Crossing the minefield

Establishing safe passage through the sensory chaos of autistic spectrum disorder

Crossing the minefield

Establishing safe passage through the sensory chaos of autistic spectrum disorder

Phoebe Caldwell

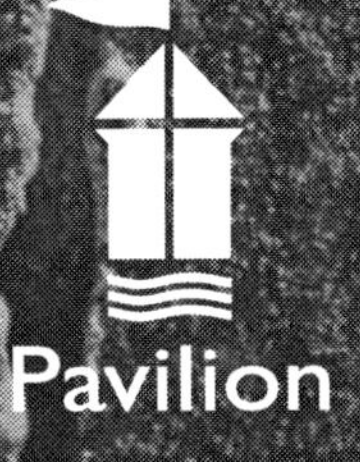

Crossing the minefield

Establishing safe passage through the sensory chaos of autistic spectrum disorder

Published by:
Pavilion Publishing (Brighton) Ltd
The Ironworks
Cheapside
Brighton
East Sussex BN1 4GD

Telephone: 01273 623222
Fax: 01273 625526
Email: info@pavpub.com
Web: www.pavpub.com

First published 2003.

A Catalogue record for this book is available from the British Library.

ISBN 1-84196-123-X

Pavilion is the leading training and development provider and publisher in the health, social care and allied fields, providing a range of innovative training solutions underpinned by sound research and professional values. We aim to put our customers first through excellent customer service and good value.

Editor: Catherine Jackson

Typesetting and layout: Jigsaw Design

Printing: Ashford Press (Southampton)

Acknowledgements

There are many people to thank, especially those who have read the manuscript and contributed ideas. Where I have used people's histories, permission has been sought except in the few cases where I have lost touch because of movements, closures and changes in providers of service. Identities have been disguised where necessary. I should also like to thank Pavilion Publishing for permission to use material from the training video *Learning the Language*.

Contents

INTRODUCTION

'Perhaps the most indispensable thing we can do as human beings every day of our lives is to remind ourselves and others of our complexity, fragility, finiteness and uniqueness.' (Damasio, 1994)

I shall start with an analogy: one that many people will still recognise. Princess Diana is promoting her campaign against landmines. A photograph, published in the newspapers worldwide, shows a fragile looking Diana crossing a minefield, following a path marked out by ribbons indicating where it is safe for her to tread. She is able to walk through this hostile environment because she knows where she is going. Neither she nor any of us would venture into such a danger zone without those guiding lines. It would be easier not to try, to stay in safety rather than to hazard our life.

This is a book about autism, or rather autistic spectrum disorder (ASD), especially – although not exclusively – where it is linked to severe learning disabilities. Its main theme is an exploration of how we can find ways to mark out a safe and meaningful progression from the isolation and sensory chaos experienced by people with ASD to relationship, by putting into the person's life points of reference that the brain will recognise and latch on to. This technique gives them confidence to move through situations that would otherwise drive them further back into their inner worlds. Furthermore, it values an individual as they are, which helps to build their self-esteem.

I have also tried to consider the affective field, the feelings that arise during interaction, and how these feelings can be employed to help both partners involved in the co-creative process into a powerful relatedness, sometimes to the level of bonding.

One of the most difficult aspects of trying to make contact with individuals who have ASD is that by the time their sensory experience is processed, it tells them that the world outside is chaotic and threatening. 'Imagine your thoughts constantly interrupted by thoughts of terror, your own voice sounding like a thunder of garbled words being thrown back at you and folks screaming at you to finish your task. People are screaming at you to stop the aggression. You find your body and voice do unusual things and you aren't in control' (Seybert, 2002). Or as Ros Blackburn, another person with ASD, put it: 'For me the whole world is a totally baffling and incomprehensible mayhem which terrifies me It is a meaningless mess of sights, sound and noise from nowhere going nowhere.' (Blackburn, 2002).

So they defend themselves by retreating to an inner world where they think they are safe.

We need to find ways to help people who are stuck in their inner world to feel safe enough to start moving out of isolation towards relationship. Like the ribbons guiding Princess Diana across the minefield, we are looking to establish guidelines, markers that the brain recognises as safe and can focus on. When we do this, the individual no longer feels they are in peril and at the mercy of their environment.

To start with, we need to ask what it is we think we are trying to achieve when we work with people with severe learning disabilities, especially those whose disabilities are linked with severe ASD or behaviour that is difficult to manage. What do we mean by a relationship with someone who may not just reject us (that would imply that they had noticed our existence) but fail even to differentiate us from our surroundings, as though we were a piece of furniture? If we try to get any closer the person may present him or herself as hostile to our presence. Is it simply that we want to find ways to contain situations that may seem to us bizarre and sometimes unmanageable? Is it that, urged on by the feeling that there must be some way to ease what may present to us as very distressful, we are looking for something more? Or is it that we see real value in each person as he or she is, and want to share our self with them in mutual exploration?

Crossing the Minefield continues the exploration of themes discussed in *Person to Person* (Caldwell, 1998) and *You Don't Know What It's Like* (Caldwell, 2000). Some of the paths may look familiar but they will take us round new corners, to see a bit further. Fresh territory is also explored. The main emphases is still on the search for what it is that has significance for this particular individual and how we can use it to bring about effective change and empower them.

Rather than starting with our own reality, it is necessary to accept that the sensory reality experienced by many people with learning disability (and/or a variety of behavioural disorders), or the interpretations that they make of their sensory intake, may present them with a completely different sensory scenario to the one that those of us without disability perceive. In particular, they may experience as scary a whole range of inputs that we see as benign. For example, a person who is deaf or who only has peripheral vision may have no warning of objects or people moving in from the side, so these present as potentially threatening because they happen suddenly and unexpectedly. The person may react in what we perceive as an aggressive manner in order to protect him or herself.

We all look at the world from our own point of view. We 'know' that 'our reality' is the true one and we respond to it in ways that correspond to our experience of it. Alternatives threaten our sense of order. Because the perception of others is different, they may react emotionally in ways that, based on our own experience, we do not expect. We find this unsettling, sometimes intimidating. It focuses our attention on the difficulties of managing their response, rather than the problems that the person is experiencing. Are we trying to cope with the effects of their behaviour rather than what is upsetting them?

Just how different the sensory reality experienced by another person may be was brought home to me by a mother who told me that her daughter, who has ASD, bites her when she tries to hug her to express her love. Naturally the mother is distressed. However we know that for some people with ASD touch is painful and that emotional expression can trigger a tidal wave of feeling. In the video *A is for Autism*, Temple Grandin describes how, as a child, she longed to be hugged, but when someone tried to do so she was engulfed by her own sensory feedback to the sensation. Instead of feeling pleasantly affirmed, she was overwhelmed. On the video this situation is illustrated by graphics of a child being swallowed up into the experience. Under these circumstances it may be that to ignore difficult behaviour in a person with ASD is to reward them – and to praise them may be experienced as punishment. What is for some of us a warm, bonding experience may be really unpleasant or even painful for someone whose sense of reality is derived from a different sensory feedback. In order to demonstrate our care and love and respect their needs, we may need to temper our own desires to express emotional closeness.

It is very easy to fall into the trap of trying to frogmarch people whose sense of reality is different from our own into the reality we know to be true for us. We may quite unconsciously project our reality onto them; we genuinely believe that what we experience is what everyone else also sees, hears and feels. My reality is real; deviations are false. But expectations, behavioural judgements and strategies based on our own sensory experience can add to the levels of stress experienced by people whose world picture is different from our own, driving them further back into their inner world. If we are prepared to learn their language so that we can enter their world, we can begin to explore what has meaning for them in ways that do not threaten them. They become interested in this non-threatening relationship and turn towards the source of a new but safe extension of their own world. We can use this approach to mark out a path between our two worlds and establish communication through processes that are meaningful to them.

Our task is to put aside our own reality and logic and keep our minds open to what is important in their world for the people with whom we work. Even where their world touches ours, we need to understand that their interpretations of situations may differ.

In the inner world, the brain and body are engaged in an internal conversation. The brain tells the body what to do and the body tells the brain it has done it. The person's focus is directed at what is going on inside them rather than making connection with the world around them. This may be because they have severe learning disability, or it may be that for one reason or another they find the outside world threatening.

Chapter One

THE USES OF SURPRISE

- Intensive interaction: getting into the brain/body language
- The 'periscope' brain
- Feeding the inner world
- Surprise as a discontinuity in expectation
- The use of surprising combinations to shift attention from the inner to the outside world

Maureen is a young woman with severe learning disabilities. She does not join in with group activities, although sometimes she will sit in on them. She is restless, preferring to stay in the corridor, where she often sits on the floor. She twists a belt or string in her hands and is distressed if this is lost.

I have met Maureen twice: once to see if I could help find ways to get in touch with her and again, ten months later, when I revisited the centre to see how she and the staff were getting on.

Maureen has a number of physical difficulties. She is mobile but leans to one side when she walks. She has a slight squint, which can make it difficult to assess whether or not she is avoiding eye contact. She hesitates when she comes to a change in floor colour, kerbs or stairs. She does not like objects coming from the side and is more able to accept them if they come from behind her. It seems likely she has tunnel vision. She has diabetes and care needs to be taken with her diet. She can become upset when her blood sugar levels are low or she has PMT or her teeth are hurting. Her behaviour reflects how she is feeling. Sometimes the reasons for her upsets are not so clear. When she is agitated she will bite her wrist, bang her head or pull her hair.

Maureen is generally non-verbal. She makes sounds and has a few words she uses occasionally. She seems to seek out the company of one particular person, a fellow user of the centre, who 'talks back' to her using similar sounds to those that she makes – they are using the same language.

Maureen has a number of characteristics that seem to come under the umbrella of autistic spectrum disorder:

- she has a number of strong repetitive behaviours
- she has an inability to form relationships
- she is inflexible, finding it hard to adapt to new situations
- she needs routines and is deeply upset by deviations from these. For example she is upset by the appearance of her mother at the centre when she is not used to seeing her there
- she is hypersensitive to some smells
- she likes her own space. This needs to be qualified as she is generally tolerant of other service users; nevertheless she does not enjoy crowded situations such as travelling on the bus. She can manage better if people sit behind her rather than in front. She does not like to be in a room with a closed door
- she does not give good eye contact and is unresponsive to interaction and attempts to relate with her
- she needs to know exactly what is happening.

Maureen responds to Intensive Interaction. This is a technique based on the primary infant/mother interaction. It uses a person's own behaviour to get in touch with them, building their movements or sounds into a 'language' that can be used to interact and hold conversations with them. The first lesson all of us learn as infants when starting to communicate is that if we do something – make a sound or movement, for example – someone will respond in a way that has meaning for us. The parent figure will confirm our utterances. Peeters (1997) says that unless we receive significant responses to our overtures we eventually give up trying. The approach known as Intensive Interaction seems to have arisen spontaneously in many countries and goes under different titles. In the UK it was initiated by Ephraim (1986) as 'Augmented Mothering', and developed as Intensive Interaction by Nind and Hewett (1994) at Harpebury Hospital School and (particularly with adults) by Caldwell (1998), and many others. It is used with people whose attention is focused on their inner world and seeks to shift their focus from solitary self-stimulation to shared activity and interaction.

The term 'Co-created Communication' is used by Nafsted and Rodbroe (1999) to describe a similar approach with deaf/blind children: 'Fluency is co-created on the level of micro-exchanges, as moment to moment adjustments.' Similarly, Nadel and Canioni (1993) describe it as: 'An on-line process of adaptation to each other within which intentions and emotions are shared and negotiated.' Rodbroe and Souriau (2000) emphasise the emotional content of the exchanges: 'Typical ways to react in a communicative way to "utterances" (an initiative by the partner which is not necessarily perceived as auditory, for example movements, pointing) is to match them by making similar movements to attune to them, by doing something which expresses that the emotional state is shared, or to imitate the contours of an utterance using another modality.'

I want to look at how this works in practice, using Maureen's history as an example.

The activities that interest and hold Maureen's attention are obvious, but to convert her transitory low-level attention into focused engagement I have to present my interventions in a way that, while partly familiar, is not quite what her brain is expecting.

My first task is to see how she is talking to herself. What feedback is she giving herself when she is self-stimulating? What is it that has significance for her in her world?

Looking at her repetitive behaviour, Maureen makes sounds and twists her belt. I find that by simply echoing these back to her I get some response. She looks up to see what I am doing.

Maureen's attention is attracted by something she recognises. As human beings we all live in a delicate balance with our environment, with everything that happens to us. From infancy we learn to respond in ways that are advantageous to us (as we see it). 'Deciding well is selecting a response that will ultimately be advantageous to the organism in terms of survival and the quality of that survival' (Damasio, 1994).

Whether or not we like it, we become biological periscopes. In the interests of survival we spend our life scanning the horizon to see if there is anything of interest. It may be an event we do not recognise and need to assess; it may be something we know is good or bad for us. In all cases our brain weighs up the situation and takes appropriate action. We are constantly on the alert. Spotting something unexpected may scare us. Our unconscious brain is notified before our conscious brain becomes aware of the danger. Two messages are sent: a fast one (the P300) to the amygdala, which prepares the body for defensive fight, freeze or flight response, and a slower one to the cortex, which weighs up the danger and if it judges there is no threat shuts down the amygdala (Greenfield, 1997).

(An example of this response occurred to me quite recently when a lorry backfired as it passed me in the road. To my surprise I found myself cowering in the hedge. I had reacted without thought to what my amygdala assessed to be a potentially threatening situation, and taken defensive action: in this case, flight. My cortex received the slower message; reassessment showed me I was in no danger and I straightened up, relaxed and laughed at myself.)

At whatever level we operate, our brain builds up a bank of images and sensations that experience has taught us require a response. As soon as we recognise one of these our brain swings into action, comparing it with previous experience and assessing its value to us. We are interested in its potential – adverse or advantageous – and this interest leads us to check up on its source. We shift our attention outwards towards events that surprise us and check them out in terms of possible benefit or threat.

Maureen recognises her sounds and looks up when she hears similar ones and when she observes me twisting a belt. However in both cases she is easily distracted by the bustle and goings-on in the busy passage.

Although it is possible to attract her attention by echoing back her behaviour, this attraction is not sufficiently intriguing to hold it. She slips back into her inner world. At this point I begin to look at other aspects of her behaviour. I have been told that she enjoys physical contact on her back, so decide to reinforce her sounds by tapping the same rhythm simultaneously on her back. This combined approach brings a very positive response. She begins to smile, laugh and watch my face to see what I will do next. She looks straight at me and repositions herself for more tapping. She becomes very relaxed and her face loses its tension. Whereas previously she had shown concern that her mother was in an adjacent room, she now walks past the room with barely a glance. After we have finished the session she spends the rest of the afternoon quietly with a member of the care staff. She does not show her usual restlessness.

When a person is locked into a repetitive loop of behaviour they are self-stimulating. In a scary or confusing world, the person knows what they are doing (Barron & Barron, 1992). The repetition soothes them and produces endorphins in the brain that feel good. Self-focus lulls them in their inner world. While they may recognise their behaviour if it is echoed back to them from an outside source, this recognition is not always enough to shift their attention from inward focus to the world outside. On occasion it may simply add feedback from the outward source to the feedback they are giving themselves. Under these circumstances the technique can reinforce the repetition. Intuitively the practitioner feels they are no longer involved in 'conversation' but are being 'used'. Far from enhancing interaction, they have become part of the furniture of the person's inner world.

The contrast between reinforcing the inner world and interacting with the world outside was particularly brought home to me during a session with Jimmy.

Jimmy is 15 and has Down's syndrome. He used to say more words but is now non-verbal apart from being able to say 'No'. He has a number of repetitive behaviours – touching his hair, ears and flipping a bundle of tickets, often so they touch his lip. He enjoys touch very much and likes to be stroked with a fibre optic strand and touched or rubbed on his back and shoulders. His moods swing and it can be difficult to predict how he will be. He can become disturbed and this behaviour makes it difficult to be with him. Recently he has started to self-harm by head banging and he can nip and pull hair. He makes sounds that change from barely audible to screaming, depending on his mood.

Jimmy likes to be in the sensory room and particularly enjoys the fibre optic lights. He will carefully choose one strand and hand it over to his care worker for them to stroke his forearm with it. He can easily use this to feed his inner world in a way that cuts out interaction. He retreats to his inner world and 'switches off'. It is as if he 'hi-jacks' objects and activities on which he is fixated and uses them to reinforce self-stimulation. This makes it difficult to communicate with him.

In this case it is not that the techniques of Intensive Interaction are at fault; rather, the approach has not been sufficiently thought through. When his arm is stroked Jimmy's brain knows what to expect and has decided that it is not worth bringing it to his conscious attention; his consciousness ignores what is familiar. We have to look for a more powerful way of attracting but also holding his attention in a sustained, focused and interactive way. We need to ask how we can make the stimulus that the person recognises more powerful and interesting than that offered by the shadows of their inner world. In practice the answer seems to be to change slightly the way in which the stimulus is presented, while retaining its general character. This can be done in a variety of ways.

Just echoing back Jimmy's sounds is not enough. To capture his attention I suggest that we echo back his sounds and simultaneously stroke his arm, using the rhythm of the sounds he makes. Whenever he makes a sound I make a movement on his arm that corresponds to the sound he has made: a short movement for a short sound, a longer one for a long sound and a wavy one for an undulating sound. We then go on to explore a number of permutations using his body language to develop interaction rather than just using the sensory equipment as relaxation. Jimmy's facial expression becomes attentive. After each movement and interaction we wait, giving him time to respond. Each time we alter the pace of the strokes to fit his sounds. He is no longer just experiencing a sensation passively but responding actively with eye contact and grinning, moving himself closer for more when asked if he wants it again. He watches my face to see what my reactions are and we maintain this mutual engagement for about an hour, until I have to end the session. His key-worker, who has known him for some years, says she has never seen him respond in this lively and engaged way before.

Working with Jimmy, there is a very strong contrast between the effect of simply joining in with his stroking and combining the stroking with his sounds: sounds that are meaningful to him, so the strokes complement them. If we return to the idea of the brain as periscope, we have introduced an additional factor: a stimulus that is sufficiently familiar because of its rhythm to be non-threatening but also different enough to be intriguing. This is interesting enough to persuade the brain to refocus on the source so that Jimmy begins to engage more deeply with the world outside.

This enhancement of the feedback a person gives himself can be done in a variety of ways.

Vicky is microcephalic. She makes a variety of sounds that can become very noisy, to the point that staff find it difficult to work in the room with her because her noises over-ride any activity they try to do. She is very cut off and they can get no eye contact. You can see she is literally talking to herself and she thinks very carefully about which of her sounds she will make next.

When I try echoing her sounds back to her through a kazoo she responds with great pleasure and makes good eye contact. She makes a sound and then turns towards me to see what I will do in response. I steer the interaction towards 'conversation'. Instead of echoing her sounds I 'answer' them. This session is filmed on video.

Watching the video later it is clear she is most intrigued when I repeat a high sound she has made and then extend it down, down, down beyond her initial utterance. As it moves beyond her initial squeal her attention becomes more acute. Her eyebrows lift, her pupils widen and darken. Her expression is almost one of disbelief: 'That's my sound but where's it going?' When I stop she turns to me and laughs. We share the joke.

Surprise is very often a discontinuity in expectation. I think I know what is going to happen within a given sequence of events, and then it doesn't, or something else does. My periscope immediately swings round to check; I start to pay more detailed attention to my surroundings in order to identify the source of the discontinuity. In practice it is 'surprise' in the context of a person's language that is critical and most often shifts their attention from their inward world to the world outside. It plays a vital role in the process of engagement. Working with deaf-blind children, Rodbroe and Souriau (2000) point out that regulating interactive play means you are always looking for ways to introduce variations to keep the interest of your partner. At the same time you have to be alert to variations suggested by your partner and respond to him or her: 'On the one hand you have to make use of repetition to create conditions that will help a deaf/blind person to have an overview and support cognitive development. On the other hand you have to add novelty to a well-known act in order not to make it dull and thereby lose the interest of your partner.'

Surprise does not always have to be in the form of an addition, something relevant added in an unexpected way. It can also arise when an anticipated event fails to happen.

Gilly has ASD and is very difficult to contact. She likes going for walks and bangs her feet on the pavement. Because there is no room to walk beside her, I follow her. Each time she treads she thumps her foot on the ground. I do the same. I have a feeling she is listening to what I am doing and this is confirmed when I deliberately miss out banging my foot. She immediately stops, turns her head and looks at me in a completely different way.

In this case it is omission that draws Gilly's attention to the world outside her inner self, but it is still a discontinuity in expectation.

Chapter Two

DRAWING BACK THE CURTAINS

- Needing to know what we are doing
- Moving on from 'games'

Ten months after I first visited Maureen, the manager of the centre tells me there has been a vast improvement in her behaviour. He describes it as though 'someone has drawn back the curtains for her'.

The set-up of the centre is a little unusual in that many of its service users are elderly, from a hospital next door and not necessarily tolerant of someone whose behaviour might be seen as (and occasionally was) threatening. I decide to go again to see if it is possible to observe the changes and to tease out what has been helpful.

Staff have clearly worked very hard and there is a noticeable change in Maureen's ability to relate. Although some of her autistic features remain, the overall impression of Maureen as someone with ASD is more difficult to sustain. Although she has good days and bad days, she now presents as lively and interactive and really enjoys being with people.

Maureen responds when her name is called by looking and sometimes smiling. She will now sometimes respond to a request for a kiss or a cuddle. Her posture has changed. Her head is more often up and she is more alert, watching what is going on. She still plays with her belt in the passage but is delighted when her keyworker joins in her games. She makes better and more frequent eye contact, laughs, initiates relatedness and watches to see what response she gets.

Although she still finds change difficult, she is more flexible and has been introduced to a number of new activities. She is not so rigid about activities always having to take place in the same location. She no longer gets upset if she has to travel on a different bus to the one she is used to. She does not have to be in the same room to eat her dinner and has learned to wait for her meal.

Her behaviour at meals is also greatly improved. Under guidance she can eat her meal with a spoon instead of shovelling food in with her hands. She no longer tears open sandwiches to eat the contents but eats the whole sandwich if it is offered in quarters. She attacks people less often. In response, other service users understand her better and are kind to her. The only user she is likely to grab is one elderly person, who is the most intolerant of her.

The major difference is that the staff now feel much happier about their interactions with Maureen. They use her sounds and body language to have fun with her. She has a particularly good key worker who enjoys 'talking' to her. She responds joyfully and her whole demeanour has changed. It is much easier to get her to come to the toilet and go for walks. They use her sounds with her, banging when she bangs, playing ball. Requests are accompanied by simple gestures to let her know what is going to happen. However Maureen is very literal. Simply pointing to the garden to indicate going out for a walk is not enough to allay her fear of the unknown. Staff first point outside and say: 'We are going for a walk …', then point to where she is standing and say, '… and we are coming back here again'. This seems to reassure her that she will be returning to a known safe place and there is now no difficulty in getting her to go outside. (These days I believe the staff don't always remember to do this but Maureen is so much more alert and relaxed that she picks up what is happening more easily.) Her key-worker says that introducing her to new things also takes less time and it only needs one person to take her out, instead of two. Also Maureen will now play a social game, responding to hiding and reappearing.

Maureen does still have off days, which may well relate to how she feels physically.

There is still work to do. For example, she looks anxious when her key-worker has to leave her temporarily. She needs to know what is happening and (as with helping her understand that she is not only going for a walk but returning to a place she feels safe) it is better to show her by gesture that you are leaving her but you will be returning.

In the middle of a game with her I am called away. I tell her where I am going and point in that direction. I then say I am coming back and point to the ground beside her. She nods and her face clears at once. For Maureen it is absolutely imperative that she knows what is going on because she feels totally threatened and abandoned otherwise.

It is critical for us to realise how serious a matter this is. If a person is unsure about what is happening, when something unexpected occurs they may quite literally feel their life is threatened. Under these circumstances the brain calls into play all the defence mechanisms we have developed throughout our evolutionary history to protect us when we think we are in mortal danger. We have to understand the degree of fear that may be motivating the person and take steps accordingly to modify our behaviour so it doesn't appear to them to presage imminent catastrophe. Helping the person understand what is going to happen allows them time to prepare for the event, to take part in their life rather than it being a lurching sequence of unpredictable and therefore scary situations. With Maureen it pays to take it slowly, breaking down each activity into small steps and getting her agreement to each before proceeding to the next.

When a person starts to come out of their inner world they may respond joyfully to 'games' based on their own body language. The danger comes if a game begins to have its own 'rules', to define itself. The process and end become predictable; the brain knows what to expect and lapses into a repetitive process. There is nothing to renew the person's focus on interaction. Instead of being an open-ended arena of potential growth, the game becomes a fixed process with no outcome. For staff also, it becomes something they have learned to 'do' with the person. Feeling themselves trapped in a situation that no longer involves exchange and has become a ritual, they will frequently ask, 'What do we do next?'

The danger of 'games' is that both parties become locked into certain ways of responding to each other. Apart from anything else, it is such fun to be able to 'respond' and get responses from someone with whom you have never been able to make contact before that there may be little incentive to try to move on. This is particularly so if neither side offers 'new' material. We know what works, and it is less demanding and safer for both parties to stay with a familiar way of enjoying each other rather than attempt to move on to unfamiliar territory. Unfortunately, if the brain is not confronted with 'new' material it can lapse into incorporating the games into self-stimulation.

This is not to say that games do not have their place, because this is when we learn to trust each other. In new situations we are vulnerable and trust is vital. Any move to incorporate unknown material represents threat, in the sense that its potential dangers have not been assessed. If we do not trust each other the interaction closes down, leading away from communication.

With Maureen it is time to move on from playing games with her to a deeper form of engagement. When I am with her I start to respond to her in ways that, while they respect her language, also contain an element she is not expecting. When her noises are placed in conjunction with touch (which is related through rhythm), she is able to use a second sense (feeling) to double check on the sound.

I also increase the interval I leave before expecting a reply from her, to give her time to think about my response, which is a little different to the one she is anticipating as she has got used to copying games. I show her keyworker how to do this and we observe how Maureen becomes quieter and more thoughtful when engaged in this type of interaction, looking at us and really thinking before she replies. She begins to initiate. At one stage she nods her head and is really pleased when we nod back, doing it again and watching carefully to see if we will answer. Instead of feeding her inner world she has shifted her focus to what is happening in the world around her. She has learned that if she nods her head she can get a response from us. It is not just about control; it is also about sharing. She has found a way of sharing in our world and is beginning to let us into hers. We can begin to explore each other in an open-ended situation.

Human beings are sentient; we have feelings, and we feel closest to people who empathise with our feelings, who understand us – even if it is understanding that we feel bad and want to be left alone. We tread on each other's feelings at our peril; this is a quick route to a broken relationship. We also let others know what our feelings are not only by how we describe them but also through our body language, which may reflect how we feel even though we are trying to conceal it.

If a person is more able, it may be that what their brain recognises is not just a reflection of its dialogue with the body but also patterns of thought and persistent themes that have been part of the conversation that the brain has with itself. For our interventions to be meaningful to them, we have to get into their mind-set.

Bob has absolutely no idea where he is in relation to his surroundings. He is fascinated by football. His keyworker has the inspiration to describe to him where things are by locating them on a football pitch: 'Look in the penalty area.' Bob finds this direction perfectly intelligible.

Lizzie's ability is overlaid by severe anxiety. She has an interest in tv soaps. Her brain very easily links up the wrong messages so she 'gets the wrong end of the stick'. We need to try and explain to her that sometimes our brain tells us things that are not true. She is unable to grasp what we are saying until it is explained in terms of an episode of Eastenders she saw. She is able to understand a complicated idea through a second-hand scenario. She does not have to think about it in relation to herself, where it threatens to overwhelm her, but can visualise it as happening in a familiar programme she has watched. Once she has grasped the concept she can move on. Another step has been taken up the ladder of understanding.

There is a footnote to the history of Maureen. Just before going to press I received an unexpected letter from her keyworker. She writes of the progress that has been made:

'Maureen seems more confident and is generally accepted with other service users now. Everybody speaks to her and passes the time of day with her. The barriers are down. She stands at the back door waiting for the clients to come in and all members greet her when they enter the building, which is nice. She seems more relaxed now and likes to be included in various activities.'

The accompanying photograph shows Maureen seated in a group at a table, turning towards a friend. Her facial expression is lively, open, alert, even radiant as he leans slightly towards her. It is her birthday and they seem to be sharing a joke.

Chapter Three

CROSSING THE MINEFIELD

- Finding the way in
- Ribbons across the minefield – using a person's 'language' to let them know what they are doing
- Reducing the hypersensitivities
- Distressed behaviour

Speaking during the plenary session of a recent conference on Intensive Interaction, a young teacher said: 'We can change people's lives.' There was a groundswell of assent from the 160 delegates present, most of them practitioners, many of them teachers in schools. The confidence with which these words were spoken is a far cry from the situation even 15 years ago, particularly for those working with adults, when the deputy manager of a large hospital wrote: 'We do not want an interactive approach in this service.'

Clearly attitudes have changed. One of the reasons is the closure of the large, long-stay hospitals. With the setting up of small group homes it has become less easy simply to warehouse people whose behaviours present management problems or who are very withdrawn. In small houses we are physically and psychologically too close to each other to ignore difficult behaviours; the movement for normalisation and age appropriateness has in many ways improved the way people with learning disabilities are perceived. Yet there is still a core of people for whom neither an improved environment nor more compassionate care nor behavioural training has provided a solution to their isolation and behavioural distress.

It is only recently that we can begin to feel that, yes, we can work effectively with these people, so many of whom shelter under the umbrella term 'autistic spectrum disorder'. Apart from changing techniques there has been a revolution in the way we think about what people with disability are experiencing. Previously, where it has been considered at all, the assumption has been that we have a common experience, that in sensory terms it's a level playing field. On the contrary, this level playing field turns out to be a whole range of mountainous landscapes. We have had to learn to recognise the validity of alternative ways of seeing things: not just 'my way is right and yours is wrong' but developing understandings of worlds that may present totally different levels of threat, triggering defence mechanisms that result in the behaviours we find challenging.

The shift has also been one of empathy, from 'training' and 'control' to motivation.

My own understanding has deepened so I now see more clearly what I am trying to do. I started out working as a helper in a department of occupational therapy in a large hospital for people with learning disabilities. It was my job to look after a group of mainly non-verbal men whose behaviours ranged from throwing furniture at each other to more personal assault. They would sit at two rows of desks with a box of beads or a clothing catalogue each, which they thumbed through. They were clearly bored. My job was to keep them quiet. Self-preservation suggested I look for some way of motivating each one of them, something they might enjoy. This led to the construction of 'games' based on whatever I could find that interested them.

Roy liked trains so I sat beside him with a fretsaw and cut out the pieces of a jigsaw of a steam engine in a station. He took the pieces one by one as they were cut off and fitted them together. We made many such puzzles. He became progressively more gentle until one day this man, who previously had been hitting people and thrusting his arms through windows several times a week, came in clutching a red rose bush he had uprooted from a garden. Blood poured over thorns as he presented it to me. It was the most touching bouquet I have ever received. (The gardener from whose flowerbed the plant had been uprooted took a rather different view.)

Together the men and I painted the walls of the corridor that formed our day room with life-sized scenes that related to their lives.

Charlie had been brought up in a pub. The bar was so life-like that Charlie tried to pull himself a pint. He also placed his ear against the landlady's chest to listen to her heart.

Fred told me his Dad had been a greengrocer. By his desk we made a shop. We painted bricks and stuck them on. We made boxes of fruit and veg. He started to tell me about his day-to-day life in the shop – an achievement, since he had very slow and limited speech.

In retrospect some of the equipment was perhaps not age appropriate. For example Jack, who had movement in only one arm, used it to lob heavy objects down the corridor, with considerable accuracy. I diverted his attention by making him a windmill that ran very smoothly on a skateboard bearing. He loved it; with it he found a better use for his one hand and sat there rocking and twirling and making happy sounds. At the time it bought us some respite. However not only was this undoubtedly a toy; perhaps more importantly, I now realise that I was feeding his inner world rather than encouraging communication. Later on his care team realised that he loved any form of transport so they took a series of photographs of him standing, getting onto or riding on different lorries, cars, motor bikes etc. This made it begin to be more possible to hold his interest in the outside world.

If we want to help people communicate and take an interest in the world outside the inner world in which they are locked we must not just use objects or activities they like to do by themselves – which may feed their inner sensations – but rather those that we can share in open-ended exploration. At the same time they must be objects or activities that the brain recognises as non-threatening so that their deployment does not drive the person back into him or herself. In a reality system that is sensory chaos the activities we offer a person are going to have to act as waymarks across the minefield, so that the person feels safe doing them. Then we can begin to use them as vehicles for interaction and extend the range of their interests.

To make quite clear what I mean by this I shall refer back to the history of Roger (Caldwell, 2000).

Roger is autistic. He attends a large and, inevitably at times, noisy day centre, almost the worst environment against which to effect improvement. He wanders round the day centre in a world of his own. He is disturbed by other service users and hits out at them if they come too near. He has quite frequent serious outbursts and is unable to take part in activities or even to go out on the centre bus. Roger makes a variety of small sounds and has a few words.

Roger's team tried out a number of approaches. Initially, they found him so exhausting that they tried working in two-hour shifts. There was no improvement in his behaviour. Reflecting on this, they saw that the constant turnover of staff might be stressful to him (just as working with him was for staff). Management used this insight to help staff understand the nature of the stress that Roger was experiencing. With management support the team switched to working with him all day and found the consistency this provided, combined with other strategies such as Intensive Interaction, using his sounds with him all the time in combination with verbal language where appropriate, was beneficial. His outbursts started to reduce.

The use of these combined approaches has made it possible for Roger to begin to relate to people – not only to his team but also to other service users – in a more friendly way. He clearly does not feel so threatened by them and may smile if they call his name. With his team he can go on the centre bus with another service user. On a good day he can go out to lunch in a pub. At the centre, serious recorded disturbances have dropped from 14 a week to one every six weeks (averaged over six months).

During this period staff focused not so much on teaching him how to do things but on how to be with him and communicate with him. Roger always had a few words but began to use a wider range in an appropriate way. A major achievement was being able to say 'Coke' to the barman, hand over his money and wait for his change. However, in spite of progress in his ability to relate and make use of appropriate words, the team continued to use his sounds to keep in touch with him. In a world that he still perceives as chaotic, keeping the link open is vital.

For Roger what was needed to effect positive alteration in his life (which resulted in improved behaviour) was the introduction of what might be termed a predictable protective shield. This acted as a buffer zone, insulating him from externally generated sensory overload and internally generated emotional overload. The 'buffer zone' provided a recognisable secure haven in which he could interpret the sensory and emotional input he received, even in the difficult environment where he lived. Because he was now held together within familiar structure – and language was used in a form he could process – he knew what is going to happen. Staff could keep in touch by responding to his sounds – sounds that were not inappropriate in a public context. All the outsider would see was an occasional murmured conversation between friends. This progress, which was achieved through the work of committed staff and good leadership, was the outcome of looking deeply at the underlying difficulties Roger was experiencing.

At this stage there was a change of leadership and because Roger was showing little sign of disturbed behaviour the special interventions were reduced, including the daily use of his language. In effect, everything he recognised was withdrawn. The effect was immediate and disastrous. He returned to his previous chaotic behaviour. Retraining the team restored the situation to one where his language was used with him and his challenging behaviour disappeared once more.

People whose sensory world is in chaos need points of reference that are intelligible to them, onto which their brain can latch. Like ribbons marking a path across a minefield, these tell them where they can safely venture. If we remove these indicators, we plunge them back into a world that is inherently unstable and may be perceived as life-threatening.

To return to the hospital and the group with which I first worked, five of the 11 men who had previously been non-verbal started to use some words appropriately. There were fewer outbursts and a marked improvement in behaviour. I now understand the basis of this approach as working through things that have meaning for the particular individual.

There are some people whose lives are totally disordered. This is reflected in behavioural outbursts that make it difficult to find care staff willing or able to look after them. One such person is Sidney.

Sid has ASD. He is extremely disturbed. He attacks staff, head butting, hitting and pulling hair. After breakfast he returns to his room, bangs his head against the wall and screams. Sometimes this will last all day. As with a number of people with ASD, his sleep pattern is disturbed and he will scream in the night. A number of staff report that he responds badly to people and crowded, demanding places.

Sid likes hot drinks frequently and some of his behaviour seems to centre around not being able to ask for them in an appropriate way.

I tried using Intensive Interaction with Sid, using his own body language to engage his attention in way that had meaning for him. In Sid's case the way his brain and body talk to each other is through touch. He strokes his face with his hands and makes sounds. These escalate as he becomes more distressed.

When I first saw Sid he was in the dining area. I sat with him while he had a cup of tea and used my hands to stroke my face and chin in the way that he was using his. He noticed fairly quickly and watched, looking at me sideways to see what I would do. When he realised that if he made a movement I would respond, he smiled.

After breakfast Sid went upstairs, following his normal pattern of behaviour, which was to shut himself in his bedroom. He became very disturbed, shouting and banging himself. I stood outside in the passage and 'answered' each of his sounds with a softer call. At first he seemed a bit confused by this but then started to come out and check whether I was still there, particularly when he heard the door at the end of the passage slam. It sounded as though I had left and he shot out to check on me. I went on using his sounds – and, when he came out, his movements. Eventually he went downstairs and into the sitting room. I stood in the downstairs passage at right angles to the room, where he could hear but not see me, and continued with his sounds. (The house manager sat at the top of the stairs and could see his responses.) It took a little while but his noises gradually subsided. At one stage he banged his head on the door – but not violently – and each time referred back to me, to see what I made of it. Each time he did this I hit the wall, but not too loudly. I particularly used a kind of sh-shushing sound he made through his fingers. In the end he went into the front room and sat down, completely calmly, by himself. For at least half-an-hour he was calm and attentive to our interaction. This intimate attention was also felt by the team leader who was observing, to the point where she felt annoyed when she was interrupted.

At this point, I made the mistake of seeing if he would tolerate my going into the room with him to work in a closer proximity. (In fact I heard the intuitive voice warning me that it was too soon to try but allowed it to be over-ridden by the practical difficulty that my time was limited.) His sounds rose and he became disturbed. However, even when he attacked a member of staff she said he was easier to disengage than normal. After he had

had a cup of tea he went up to his room and made no more sounds for another half hour while we were there. His house leader said this was unusual.

It was clear from Sid's response that Intensive Interaction offered the possibility of getting through to him in a way that staff had not found possible up until now. Guidelines given to the staff team reminded them that it was very important to get the spacing and timing right. Particularly, they should not hurry him but give him time to think and to respond. They should be careful not to 'hype him up', always aiming to calm him and paying careful attention to the emotional content of his sounds, letting empathy sound in their replies. While it was important at times to have fun with him, when he was distressed they needed to learn to 'stay with' his upset.

Two weeks later his team leader reported that Sid was getting better and responding to her team's use of his 'language'. He now touched her head to say, 'Goodbye': a personal gesture that he had not been able to make before.

If people with autism are upset it is because they cannot handle the amount of sensory input they are getting. When it is too much they get overloaded. The images, sounds and other sensory feedbacks, both from their inner and outer worlds, break up. This is a process known as fragmentation, which also involves confusion and sometimes severe physical pain. A small boy complains his head is going 'fuzzy', another that his head is 'going away'. Lindsey Weekes, interviewed in the Radio 4 programme A Bridge of Voices, described how, when he became sensorily overloaded as a child, he would crash his head against the wall or run in front of a car – anything to stop the pain.

Not only do we need to use a person's language so that we can share their lives; we also need to look at what triggers what is, in many cases, a manifestation of extreme distress, which is how I interpreted Sid's disturbances. However most people with ASD do seem to devise coping strategies that they learn to use as they grow up, to protect themselves from too much sensory overload. Such strategies fall roughly into two groups:

a. repetitive behaviours that produce endorphins (the feel-good factor). Also, in a world of sensory chaos, they let a person know what they are doing and provide a point on which to focus so they do not have to listen to what is going on around them. More able people may focus on themes such as particular videos or interests, rather than bodily sensations. These become part of the furniture of their inner world and we call them fixations

b. exit strategies that remove the person from the source of their discomfiture in one way or another. (For example this might include physically removing him or herself from the source of discomfort, gaze avoidance, shutting eyes, or attacking people so they will go away.)

However there are some people, and I think Sid is one of them, who seem to have been unable to develop effective defences to protect themselves, even when they are adult. When we looked at his environment with this in mind, it was clear that the dining area was extremely noisy at breakfast: a lot of people, some of whom were also disturbed, milling around in an unpredictable fashion in a small area to the extent that I also felt the pressure. I suggested the team should look for some way of offering him a more tranquil environment.

The team leader suggested he should be taken to MacDonald's for breakfast, to get him out of the house until the other residents had left for their daytime activities. You might think this would also be a potentially threatening environment but it is quiet at that time of day and there is another important difference: the local McDonald's is not personally invasive; no one trespasses on the privacy of his inner world in way that distresses him; it does not impinge on his private space in the same way as the hurly-burly of his home territory.

This combined approach of using Sid's language, plus reducing the environmental impact he finds so difficult, seems to be working very well. His team still have some problems but overall they describe his behavioural difficulties as very much improved.

We need to change the way we perceive people with severe behavioural disorders so that when we are considering strategies, what we have uppermost in our mind is the sensory difficulties with which they are struggling, rather than the outbursts we find so hard to manage. For this reason it may be better to think in terms of 'distressed behaviour' rather than challenging behaviour (a term that, while it was introduced originally to describe behaviours that challenge the system, is now widely used to describe behaviours that present a personal challenge to staff). This can lead to care staff feeling endangered before they even start, by a reputation that should more rightly direct us to the inability of an individual to handle the distress they are experiencing.

At the end of a visit to Mike, who has severe distressed behaviour, his house leader says to me: 'Always before people have come and tried to tell us how to change him. No one has suggested before that we need to change ourselves.'

Chapter Four

WE DIDN'T BELIEVE YOU

- Using a person's language to reduce distressed behaviour

'When you said that if we learned to use Reg's language with him, learned to talk to him through his sounds and movements, his difficult behaviour would diminish, we went away and laughed. We didn't believe you. However, we did it because we were told to and that is precisely what happened.'

The speaker was a young care worker at a meeting to discuss how life had changed for Reg – and the people who looked after him, since an original intervention two years previously.

Reg is 22 and lives in a separate flat in a community home. His behaviour presents as falling within the autistic continuum. He avoids eye contact. He routinely 'touches' walls and surfaces, continuously checking on his space, probably trying, as Jolliffe puts it, to work out the pattern of what is happening and reassuring himself as to where things are.

When I was first asked to see him Reg's reputation for negative behaviours was such that I doubted very much whether I could help. He spent a lot of his time in his room, shouting and self-injuring violently, which would extend to attacking staff who tried to intervene. He would wander about naked. On occasions he would become agitated and strip off in public places without warning. Sometimes it was possible to assign causes to his outbursts – at others the reasons were untraceable. It had reached the stage where staff admitted they were scared to come to work, scared of him and particularly scared that they would not be able to cope with him in public. They said they rarely got through a day without incidents. Often these were prolonged and difficult to handle.

Remember, in sensorily chaotic surroundings a person who uses a repetitive behaviour knows what they are doing. People with ASD maintain their sense of coherence in a multitude of different ways. Donna Williams, in her book *Somebody Somewhere* (1994), describes how, as a child, 'she would search the eyes looking back in the mirror, looking for meaning, looking for something to connect with'. In the Radio 4 programme A Bridge of Voices, Lindsey Weekes describes how people with ASD at a disco will focus on the strobe lights to cut out the sensory chaos. For a number of people, it seems that the sensation of 'feeling in the sense of touch/holding' may not break up when the other senses do. For example, another person with autism, Gunnilla Gerland describes how, when she heard the sound of a moped, all sense of a coherent environment broke down so that she was unable to distinguish up and down. In order to maintain some sense of coherence she would cling to iron railings. At least she could feel something stable (Gerland, 1996).

A man keeps a clothes peg on his finger; at least he can feel that. A child asks for his fluffy pig when he is becoming upset. Holding something their senses recognise lets these people know what they are doing at a time of sensory breakdown.

Each of these people is reaching for a sensation to which they can cling in order to maintain some sense of stability when everything else is falling apart.

Reg's communication is limited although he has a few 'words' that are his private sounds for different objects. If he is happy to let you touch him and feels safe in his surroundings he will reach out his hand and say 'mop', but apart from this he is unable to communicate effectively. He is always fixated on something, particularly the colour of his shirts and sweaters, although the favoured colour changes from time to time.

To distract him his key worker used to 'draw' with him, but not in way that was interactive. Engagement was mechanical – Reg getting other people to do the drawings. If prompted he would hand over the pens he wanted his key worker to use, but showed little interest in the process, looking round in other directions. He would spend a considerable amount of time taking the 20 or so essence and coloration bottles from the shelf in the kitchen cupboard and lining them up on the work surface. When he had identified them all, he replaced them. Attempts at diversion did not work and distressed him. It was impossible to interrupt him. Observation suggested his activities were actually a way of keeping people at bay rather than engaging with them.

Reg also has a number of sounds and body and facial movements, such as hands to the mouth and clicking. These activities have real meaning for him and express how he is feeling. (Staff say of his sounds or gestures, 'That is a happy sound/gesture – that is stressed'. It is possible to tell how Reg is feeling by observing his body language.) When these are echoed back to him and used as a framework to 'talk' to him he will begin to give real and interested eye contact.

Using a person's own language, it is often possible to work with their self-injurious behaviour. The one time Reg hit his chest when I was with him (which was when the hall in the centre was particularly noisy) I smacked mine and continued to do so at intervals. He stopped trying to hit himself and his interest focused on me. He held out his hand and said, 'mop'. I had the feeling we were in empathy with each other. (This technique was also tried successfully by Jim, his keyworker.)

Meeting two years later with the team leader and staff involved, we discussed the changes in Reg's life and what it had meant for the people working with him. Jim said that the introduction of an interactive approach, both in terms of using his sounds and touching Reg's hands as conversation – and also in using all his activities as opportunities for sharing – had led to them communicating with Reg on his terms in a relaxed, low-key way. (They are careful not to hype him up but rather make sure they keep the interaction quiet and centred.) Previously they had been trying to 'manage' and 'control' Reg's life; they were telling him what to do. In particular they felt they were trying to teach him skills in a way that was actually increasing his stress levels and hence the levels of disorientation he was experiencing, driving him back into his inner retreat. Now they were sharing activities, doing them together. They felt they had a different model for the relationship and were much more laid back and responsive. They started with his agenda rather than their own, making fewer demands on him.

Another member of staff who used to work with Reg but had not seen him for some time said she could not believe the difference – not only the reduction in his distressed behaviour but also the increase in his general responsiveness. When she returned for an occasional shift, she soon slipped into a 'conversation' with him. He began to test how far she could manage, eventually taking his sounds up to a high squeal. She reacted quite spontaneously, throwing up her hands and laughing: 'I can't manage that', and he burst out laughing with her.

This may sound a small incident but it marks the change from an isolated, unhappy life to one where initiating and sharing fun and jokes is possible. It highlights the change in his quality of life. Previously staff viewed his noises and body language as something that Reg should be distracted from, so the message he got was that the activities that had meaning for him were not important. Now people listen to his communications and take notice of what he wants to do. He is a valued and more self-confident person, with control of his situation.

Reg's care staff soon forgot to be self-conscious. (Some people do find this difficult initially, particularly if the person they are working with is banging himself or an object, as the instinct is to restrain him. In practice the brain is surprised to hear its rhythm coming from elsewhere and the person almost always stops and listens, which gives us a chance to break into the inner cycle in which they are locked when we respond to them in an empathetic way.) The staff soon found that using his language became a matter of course throughout the day; they did not wait until there was a crisis to deal with. In public they just use small sounds so that it does not draw attention to him as 'different'.

Outbursts are a rarity. If they do occur staff feel confident to go into his room and deal with them, which previously they were reluctant to do. Because Reg also feels more confident as an outcome of interaction, he has begun to initiate activities himself. One day he was with his key worker, Jim, who was using his language with him. He became very relaxed and happy. Later, when he needed to get dressed, Jim offered him his pants, which he threw back. Instead of pushing the issue, Jim continued in his language. In a little while Reg got up and dressed of his own accord. On another day he and Jim were watching a video. He suddenly got up and went and loaded the dishwasher without any prompting. If he comes down in the morning before dressing, he wears his pyjamas instead of coming down naked. Situations that would have triggered outbursts no longer do, even those that are stressful. At a football match the ball was accidentally kicked hard into his chest. After an initial surprise reaction, he settled back quite calmly to watch.

In spite of what we may instinctively feel, it is not disrespectful to engage with people through their own language; on the contrary. Donna Williams, in the Channel 4 film Jam-Jar: An Inside Out Approach, talks about the terrible strain of always having to talk and be in 'their world', in a world where alien sounds have to be interpreted into meaning. It is important that we do not judge what is meaningful for the people with whom we work by what is meaningful for us.

Chapter Five

OVER AND OVER AGAIN

- The use of repetitive behaviours
- How Intensive Interaction can keep the brain-body conversation open-ended

Infant initiates, parent confirms and the infant moves on. When we are little we are faced with experiencing everything and comprehending nothing. We are the experiences that happen to us. To survive, we wrestle to bring order out of chaos; finding worlds we cannot control, we struggle to create those we can. For example, our infant brains repeatedly tell us to wave our fingers or say a sound until we receive confirmation of our activity. We test our sensations on our senses – when we feel 'waving our fingers', they move, and vice versa. We double check on our external references – our parents, who copy back to us what we do, confirming our activities. We continually repeat the action until we are satisfied we know what will happen when we perform a particular action. We go on until we are sure the pattern is established – a benign form of perseverance. At this stage the brain moves on to give the body another set of instructions. The trigger for the 'switch-off' is very specific: the recognition that the particular message sent by the brain to the body produces a recognisable response in our body in terms of its activity. This is the way we have all learned what we are doing.

Ideally, a dyadic relationship is set up between mother or mother figure and infant. In this game, the infant initiates a sound or behaviour – for example, 'Boo' – and the mother or parent figure echoes it back until the infant's activity is sufficiently confirmed and it goes on to something else. The mother suddenly realises the baby is no longer on 'Boo' but has moved on to 'Da'. This is the pattern of reality testing and one of the means by which communication is established and the baby learns. It is also a form of repetition that the baby switches out of once it has established a particular pattern. Either the brain turns off the message or, judging it to be of little importance, we stop listening to it. But what if for some reason, the switch-off mechanism fails?

Gunnilla Gerland tells us: 'I had no natural brake inside me' (Gerland, 1996).

I want to look at what happens when individuals are caught up in repetitive behaviours where for one reason or another the brain is failing to switch off. Such people have become stuck in a groove, with the brain continuously sending the same message over and over again. This may be because at the time they were born the brain was not ready to 'play' the exploration game. By the time the brain had matured enough to do so, the parent had given up trying, so the switch-off mechanism does not develop because the brain never gets a meaningful response. Alternatively, it may be that the switch-off mechanism does develop and then fails. Either way we are left with a brain that, instead of talking to the world outside, talks to itself.

Temple Grandin's description quoted earlier of the discomfort caused by her hyper-sensitivity to touch also illustrates the inability of her brain to terminate the feedback from her body. 'If you put on a pair of scratchy pants and then take them off, that is the end of your discomfort, but if I wear scratchy pants and take them off, a fortnight later I am still experiencing that discomfort.'

I had always considered this anecdote in terms of the experience of discomfort until one day I was thinking about perseverance and realised that what Grandin was actually talking about was the inability of her brain to switch off the feedback she was getting from her body. This led me into further speculation about the nature and origins of repetitive behaviour.

As pointed out previously in *You Don't Know What It's Like* (Caldwell, 2000), we all have repetitive behaviours: breathing, for example. I also paid tribute to the extraordinary account by Donna Williams in *Nobody Nowhere* (1992) of the evolution of a repetitive behaviour, moving from her early fascination with coloured flecks in the air through to a fixation with glass beads. The question is, whether or not we are focusing on these behaviours, are we conscious of what we are doing? During our childhood we explore particular objects or activities with all the tenacity of full-blown fixations. We become linked into a particular physical sensation or feeling or activity. We begin to investigate its possibilities, playing with it in our minds in ways that 'progress beyond simple investigation of the physical sensations it arouses, to a process which can allow us to explore our anxieties and understand the world around us' (Moyles,1989).

Playing with feelings allows us to adjust as we make the transition from dependence on the mother to what Winnicott calls the 'insult of reality'. He points out that, if weaning is successful in psychological terms, as the mother withdraws her breast and reality impinges the child develops a third space, a transitional space that is a parallel world, neither 'me' nor 'not me', a sort of testing ground where they cut their new experiences down to manageable size. 'This third part of the life of a human being is an intermediate one of experiencing, to which to which inner reality and external life both contribute' (Winnicott, 1971).

It is here, in this free-floating pre-integrative space, before everything has been fully taken on board and ordered, that the child learns to cope by dealing creatively with anxiety through games and simulated scenarios, modifying and improving its understanding. For all of us, this is a journey that helps us bring meaning to our circumstances. We call it play: through it we learn to make sense of our senses and the feedback our senses initiate.

If we are lucky, that is; it does not always happen like this. 'Of every individual who has reached the stage of being a unit with a limiting membrane and an inside and an outside, it can be said there is an inner reality to that individual, an inner world that can be rich or poor, at peace or in a state of war' (Winnicott, 1971).

If we encounter an outside world that we perceive as totally hostile or chaotic, the only way that we can build a world we can control is through and in our inner world. Instead of focusing on the world about us we give up and retreat to a world that is unassailable. We start to take refuge in the sensation for itself and can become trapped, revisiting it again and again. The object or feeling becomes an end in itself. In the film Jam Jar, Donna Williams describes her disastrous childhood – the demands she could not meet and the failure of those around her to understand her world: 'All that created a war in me and I went back into my world.'

Either we learn to range freely in our world through creative exploration or we retreat. Sometimes both possibilities can co-exist. This is illustrated in the following history of one small boy, as told me by his mother. In particular his story explores a movement out of a potentially closed behavioural pattern to an open-ended resolution through the medium of his mother's intuitive assessment of the child's motivation. Confirming the meaning of his play she allows him to move on. I quote it with her permission.

Doug has ASD. At the age of three he was holding on to his bowel movements until he was in bed. He then smeared himself – a messy business that left him and his plastic animal toys and bedclothes covered with faeces. This happened repeatedly until the community nurse suggested regulating his movements with senna, so that he would have to release them during daytime. One evening before the new regime of medication was started, his mother was late bringing the washed animals to him in bed. As soon as she brought them, Doug passed his motion and proceeded to dip their faces in the stool, making mouthing sounds. His mother realised that Doug was feeding them. When she gave Doug coco pops as a substitute, the smearing ceased and did not recur.

If we use the criteria of our world, how easy it is to mis-assign motivation.

However, there is another important point to this story. One of the features looked for in diagnosis of ASD, along with the level of communication and ability to relate, is the question of whether the child is capable of imaginative play. Doug deals with anxiety through an activity that is clearly rudimentary play, no different from any other child feeding his or her dolls with pretend food. He knows about feeding so he feeds his animals in the only way he has at his disposal, however inappropriate it may be deemed to be. In a world that he must have been finding chaotic in sensory terms this 'play with intent' became a way of coming to terms with an impossible situation, learning how to cope with what was happening in a way he could control. His anxiety became extremely pronounced if he was not able to follow his routine when he needed to. (This 'play' was so striking that I checked on the nature of his assessment. Was he really autistic or was there some other disability? Doug had been assessed at the age of 26 months as having ASD by a psychologist, followed by an assessment centre.)

Doug is now four. He continues to feed his animals coco pops out of a cereal bowl. However although he has other repetitive behaviours this is not one of them as it is no longer compulsive. What started as a game and looked as if it was going to become a fixation was opened out through his mother's accurate assessment of its importance and meaning for him. He still plays it sometimes, but for fun rather than under compulsion.

We know that repetitive behaviour is present in infants and is in an infant an essential part of learning. Is it possible that what we call stereotypical and fixated behaviour can, at least sometimes, start as a game but, because of a general tendency to be unable to switch off once a pattern is established in the brain (perseveration), end up as a fixation? This would imply that the capacity for imaginative play may be present initially but that perseverance takes over. What is evident is that Doug, age three with ASD, was capable of playing a 'game' that was in danger of becoming part of a repetitive cycle. Thanks to his mother's observation, the action taken by her both confirmed his behaviour and introduced a creative resolution and Doug was able to move on.

What I am suggesting is that, at least in some children with ASD, the instinct to play is present but because of adverse circumstances, which may be either internal or external, this instinct is swallowed up in perseverance: that fixations and repetitive behaviours start in the same way as games but become closed off. Intensive Interaction helps to keep games open-ended by confirming the activity and so encouraging the brain to move on in ways that are safe for that person.

Chapter Six

FINDING EACH OTHER

- Knowing where we are; getting lost in sensation
- Projection
- Where am I? Being present; finding ourselves so that we can be present to others
- An excursion into 'feeling'
- The transitional playground: what does it feel like?
- Affect
- Moving beyond disability
- Relatedness
- Where shall we meet? Being simultaneously empty and present
- The doorway of sensation

This section draws on Damasio's *Descartes' Error* (1994) and *Autism and Sensing* by Donna Williams (1998).

Where are you?

We are all engaged in three conversations running simultaneously. The 'thinker' is involved in internal messaging. Simultaneously the brain, the 'works manager', is talking to and receiving feedback from the body, while the 'negotiator' talks to the world outside. To do this we need to be able to shift our focus from our inner world and engage with the world outside. We have to change gear.

To which of these conversations am I listening? Which is uppermost in my mind? Each of us will have a different balance of attention. For example, if I am hurt I am going to pay most attention to the works manager. If I am trying to write, my brain is listening to myself; I am thinking. When I am relating to someone else my mind is on interaction, so the negotiator is uppermost, but the thinker is also present to monitor our conversation. The balance is constantly shifting according to need.

When a person finds the outside world too hostile they cease to relate to the world outside. For many of them, the works manager comes to dominate the brain's activity. They listen to and engage with the feedback they are receiving from their own bodies. For example they may listen to their own breathing rhythm, something we might only do if we were practising certain forms of yoga or meditation.

But communication is a two-way business. When a person is locked into their inner world our first task is to understand how that person is talking to herself, so we can ease into the conversation using her brain-body language. This sounds straightforward but in this section I want to consider the complexities that may arise when a person is so totally identifying with a sensation she is giving herself that, in effect, she 'becomes' that sensation. Where, for example, do I address a person whose sense of self appears to emanate from her foot, from her shoulder or even from outside herself, from a toy? How do I speak to someone who in a psychological sense seems to have moved house?

If you ask someone how they know that they are, how they know they exist, they will probably say that they 'feel' they are. Sitting on this chair I feel my feet on the floor and the seat against my legs and backside. The hardness of the wood is experienced in my flesh. I get feedback to my brain from an external source that tells me my position. Balance is called into play to keep me in an upright position so I do not fall off. At any one time I know that I am because of the feedback I get from the objects that surround me and from the secondary feedback from my own body.

It is interesting that when we receive a signal that gives us information about the world outside, our brain actually receives two signals. The first is information about the object and the second is from the sense organ that senses it, simultaneously telling the brain which sense (smell, touch, taste etc) processed the information. Learning something about an object that is outside us is accompanied by learning about our own body state.

'A special sense such as vision is processed at a special place in the body boundary, in this case the eyes. Signals from the world outside are thus double. Something you see (or hear) excites the special sense of sight as a "non-body signal" but it also excites a "body signal" hailing from the place in the skin where the special signal entered. When you see, you do not just see, you feel you are seeing something with your eyes' (Damasio, 1994).

Most of us who do not have ASD have a good idea of our body boundary. Although we do not often think about it, we know where 'I' stops and where 'the other', 'not me', begins. Information about our body state normally remains in the background unless we deliberately turn our attention to it. It is a question of where our interest is focused. Previously (Caldwell, 1998) I have described how some people with severe or profound disabilities or ASD will focus on simple repetitive behaviours such as breathing rhythms, which it would be normal for us to ignore unless we were practising some such exercise as yoga. What I am trying to bring out is that when people who do not have ASD focus on a particular activity or object, in addition to the sensory information we receive about that external object or activity, we also get information about the interface: which bit of the body is receiving the signal. So if an object is outside us and we are paying attention to it, because of the double signal (one from the object to the brain about the object and one from whichever sense organ perceives it to the brain, telling the brain that the eye or ear or skin has received the information, depending on the mode), we are also getting information about our boundaries – where in the body the signals are arriving – that is, through our eyes, ears or skin. We learn about our boundaries at the same time as we receive information about the world outside. Lack of this may be critical for a person who has very little sense of who and what they are unless they are focusing on a behaviour that is familiar. Sean Barron (1992) tells us how secure it made him feel to switch the lights on and off – 'he knew what he was doing'. It seems possible that his enhanced sense of security derived not only from being able to control at least something in a chaotic world but also from becoming conscious of his body state, knowing his boundary, being able to differentiate between himself and other, knowing who he was.

A child who bangs her head responds to her doctor who asks why she does it by saying that she does it to know she is there.

In a confusing world she needs a violent sensory stimulus that she can recognise to help her know her body state.

Janice is totally absorbed in rubbing her thumb on her fingers. This is where she 'feels herself', where she experiences her self, to the extent that when she is invited to come for a meal she fails to respond, even when prompted through an object of reference in the form of her plate and a spoonful of dinner. However when it is suggested that her thumbs might like some dinner she comes without hesitation. It is clear she has identified with the place she feels herself to be.

Janice has identified with an affect. This is where her attention is. It is only here, through the doorway of this sensation, that we will be able to make contact with her. This is where we must look.

Therapists will talk about a person being 'centred' or 'off-centre'. These are states that are difficult to describe except in intuitive terms. They relate to whether the person is truly herself as she is, or whether she is somehow mis-aligned. In some cases the person may actually relocate her sense of self to the object or sensation with which she is engaged. In extreme cases she may have identified with some other activity or person, or projected on to someone else a part of herself that she cannot handle.

Marie's only spoken language is a repetitive phrase, 'Rupert the Bear, Rupert the Bear'. It is not just that she is fond of her toy bear but more that she identifies herself with it. Like Janice, just inviting her to a meal does not get through to her. She only responds, gets out of her chair and walks to the door, when asked if Rupert the Bear would like lunch. She becomes stressed by demands she does not understand when the question is addressed to her directly. This is not where she is. It is as if the postman has delivered a letter to the wrong address.

In Marie's situation, it would be proper to understand 'Rupert' as a 'transitional object', a link object that stands between dependence on the mother and independence (Winnicott, 1971). Such adopted objects have great significance in developmental terms. To try to remove or ignore them is to cause great distress and damage, setting the person back in developmental terms. They cling to them for security. For Marie, Rupert is so important that she identifies herself with it. The way forward is through acknowledgement and attention, and through using the object as material for open-ended games.

Sometimes I am asked if it is not retrograde to 'pander' to this form of communication, whether it is not more appropriate to insist that a person responds to 'our language'. To do so would be to prioritise our reality over and above the person's ability to understand. What this really shows is a lack of understanding of the processes in which people can become trapped. The downside of this route is that, while they may understand from body language that a demand is being made of them, if the demand has no meaning for them the level of stress is increased. They may learn to conform by making signs or sounds but still not attach meaning to them, leading to disappointment and frustration when they do not get what they hoped for.

For a person with autism, very severe learning disabilities and distressed behaviour, the primary consideration should be the need for contact. Above everything else we need to establish communication; the need for this should override our worries about the way in which it is done. This is more important for them than that we are able to feel we have taught them something. The outcome of trying to frog-march people into understanding what is for them a threatening input may display itself in outbursts of distressed behaviour, however desirable the end may seem to us.

In these situations it is not just enough to know how a person is talking to herself; we also have to know where it is she feels she is, in the sense that she feels in sensory contact with herself. A good place to start looking is where or how that person is giving herself sensory stimulus. Unless we understand this, we may find we are addressing empty space.

As well as knowing where the other person is in psychological terms, it is also helpful to know where we are, so that we do not impose on and attribute to others feelings that properly belong to us. Because I know where my boundaries are and who is related to whom, I must not assume that you do.

Where am I?

Autism (and much learning disability) happens when the brain is 'not wired up properly' as Lindsey Weekes puts it in A Bridge of Voices. The aim of this section is to move beyond disability to relationship. It is trying to grapple with the essence of what it is to be me and you together – us. If this means an excursion into some rather shadowy speculation I am unrepentant, because the deeper we look into what it is that we are doing, the more we become aware of our common humanity, what it is that binds us together and what we can give to and learn from each other. I am aware that I am trying to present sometimes subtle psychological states in simple language. If the attempt opens our eyes or even helps us to look, it will be successful.

I know where I am – we all do. We have a very strong presence of self, derived from our sensory feedback that tells us where we are and what we are doing.

Or where we think we are – because, like some of the people we work with, we also may be displaced. At the simplest level, we may be physically present but not mentally alert to the situation we are in. Our attention may wander.

A key worker is observing a session of Intensive Interaction. He turns to speak to anther member of staff as they pass. While his aside is relevant, as he turns his head away he misses the moment at which Robbie starts to attend and respond – the left corner of his mouth starts to twitch at the beginning of a smile. By the time the key worker has turned back it is no longer clear which was the critical sensory stimulus that captured Robbie's attention.

We cannot afford to withdraw our attention or let it wander for a second or we may miss the one signal that tells us the key is starting to turn in the lock, when the person first begins to relate to the world outside them. We must be present for the person we are working with.

I can only speak for myself, so much of this section will be deliberately written in the first person. This is because self-scrutiny involves working with feelings – and mine is the only inner world of perception I can locate. I may surmise or presume about yours, or be inclusive by writing 'we', but with all the possible weaknesses and blind alleys that beset self-examination I cannot know what you feel in the sense of experiencing it. To talk about 'you' or 'one', to depersonalise the journey into 'it', is to move into second-hand territory. The point of this journey is to reach the centre, not only that of the person with whom I am engaged but also my own. Without this we may miss out on each other.

The word 'feeling' is a linguistic quagmire because we use the word in so many different ways. 'I feel the chair' is simple. It is a direct sensory experience – in this case touch, a response to an external stimulus. This is immediately complicated by the fact that, although I feel the chair if I turn my attention to it, most of the time I have learned to cut out this type of sensation even while it is happening, in order not to clutter myself with unnecessary stimuli. So attention is also a factor in the equation of feeling. In addition, such an experience may also be that of internal sensation: for example, balance or proprioception. 'I feel angry' describes my emotional state. It is a response, sometimes to a real external trigger, or it may be that anger has been so long the pattern of my life it has become a state and I will respond with anger to situations that would not normally demand it. 'I feel that you are angry' moves into the shadowy and subliminal world of perception where I pick up on your emotion and it triggers feeling in me. This is a danger zone because on the one hand I may be picking up your anger and on the other it may be that I cannot bear my own anger so I transfer it to you. Rather than being able to own my anger, I see it as yours: 'I feel that you are angry with me.'

Even this very brief analysis of how we use the word 'feeling' demonstrates how easy it is, in terms of language, to confuse triggers with reactions to triggers, the causes with our internal responses, the emotions with the footprints of sensation (what we are left with).

I use the term 'affect' here to describe my emotional response to a sensory experience. Thus, I feel the chair is hard: the affect is my irritation at being made uncomfortable. According to Damasio, in this sense – the sense of affect – our feelings are: '… the direct perception of a specific landscape – that of the body…they are the result of a most curious physiological arrangement that has turned the brain into the body's captive audience' (Damasio, 1994).

We learn to draw from its context the sense in which the word feeling is used. However, whichever way we choose to express it, all imply attention as well as proximity, either in the physical or the psychological sense. (I may reject a feeling but that is a matter of choice, even though the reasons for my decision may not be deemed important enough by my brain to be brought to my conscious attention. For example, my brain is aware through sensory feedback that I am sitting on a chair but has decided it is not important enough to bother my conscious mind with, unless the chair is unexpectedly tilted, in which case I am in a situation that is potentially threatening and my balance organs immediately inform me. Until the chair was tipped, my brain had made a decision based on previous experience without bothering to inform me.)

However, as best I can, I have learned that I am – and I also know that you, out there, are different from me. I have a strong feeling of my 'self', the 'me' and the 'not self', 'not me'. Although they are to some extent flexible, I know my boundaries. (If I am writing, my sense of me may include the pen that I write with. This is partly because of where the sensation is: not only the feeling on my fingers of the pen but also, beyond that, I am feeling the pressure of the pen on the paper. To take it further, when I am driving I may enlarge my sense of self to cover my car, the boundary then being my wheels and the tarmac. I may include my possessions in the feeling of self and react as if I myself am threatened if my possessions are threatened. (Under certain circumstances I may even feel threatened enough to ask what people are doing on 'my road', trying to take possession of something that is clearly not mine.)

It was not always like this. As an infant I was unable to distinguish between myself and other. I thought, or rather experienced, all the world as 'me'; I did not know there was anything else. Differentiation came slowly as I learned through exploration of the senses to distinguish myself (in this body) from other things and bodies, from the reality of out there. Certain things always responded to me – if I waved my fingers I could see the movement. I learned to test reality by double-checking through an alternative sense: in this case feeling and vision. Other things responded to me if I cried. My mother came – but not always; her attention was intermittent. Presence and absence must have been helpful in showing my self what was me.

'From the beginning the baby has maximally intense experiences in the potential space between the subjective object and the object objectively perceived, between me-extensions and the not-me. This potential space is at the interplay between there being nothing but me and there being objects and phenomena outside (my) objective control' (Winnicott, 1971).

I learned by exploring the boundaries of my control through physical sensations. Gradually I became aware not only of others but also that others experienced a different reality from mine. I learned to negotiate and compromise. Through relationships with others I came to know not just that I am but also who I am.

Donna Williams, who is high functioning, brings us remarkable insight through her books, video and film, which help us compare our experiences of differentiation with that of a person with ASD. In her book *Autism and Sensing* (1998) she describes how, in her earliest years, she accumulated experience of things outside herself in an unsorted jumble of indiscriminate sensory experiences. She talks about 'merging' and 'resonance' to describe her early relationships with objects outside herself, and continues: 'One could ask what is the experience of merging, of resonance, worth if there is none of the reflection or consciousness which comes with bringing a conscious sense of self to the experience. Perhaps only in death will I ever know again what it is to lose myself so wholly in the experience of "other" without sense of time or space, with no past or future and no here. There is no deeper experience than the total encapsulation of self within an experience until one is indistinguishable from that experience.'

This suggests a retreat to the undifferentiated perfection of the womb. Progress in differentiating herself from objects outside appears to have been uneven and difficult, progressing through a stage she calls 'mono' where she was either able to sense an object or herself but not herself in relationship to the object: 'I could not process information from the outside and inside at the same time. I was either in a state of jolting perceptual shifts, or remained in one sensory channel or the other.'

In fact she explored physical sensations without processing her bodily response to those sensations: 'Either I existed or other existed and I did not.'

She goes on to distinguish between merging, or resonating, which involve no intent, and acts where consciousness is involved: 'Trying is an act of mind and mind is consciousness and this is to have a conscious "sense of self". To merge with an object is to become it and one cannot do that with an intact sense of separate simultaneous existence...Once there is a conscious sense of self there is always separateness from other and always separability... one filters information and interprets sensory experience. This...begins to limit how we perceive something external to us. We no longer take it in exactly as it is.'

Exactly how we perceive our boundaries may also be cultural, and I recognise that my feeling of individual 'self' is personal and a part of the western experience. There are parts of the world where what I experience as 'self' is perceived as 'we'; the sense of the collective is stronger than that of the personal. I also understand that this other way of 'knowing' is just as valid as my experience, but I have to stick to my own baseline. It is worth noting, however, that the closer I am to my feeling of myself, the more available I am for others, the more I can enter the collective experience of 'we'. In Winnicott's terms, the boundary that I have perceived as a gulf between 'me' and 'other' becomes an intermediate playground, the place where my world and the world of other can overlap in a creative way and I can truly experience what is 'not me'. Put very simply, I need to be myself in order to know others and, as developmental psychologist Suzanne Zeedyke (2002) has pointed out to me, paradoxically I need to know others before I can come fully to know myself. 'We' is the path to 'I'.

Hobson puts it in terms of language: 'Consciousness is a matter not just of thinking but also of feeling. Self-consciousness (as awareness of self) involves adopting a perspective on oneself through identifying with the attitudes of others. We cannot understand the concept of "I" and "You" until we grasp the possibility of reciprocal roles in speech. It is the person who speaks who anchors meaning to the word, I. We have to grasp relationship before we can identify and think about self' (Hobson, 2002).

Winnicott (1971) lays great emphasis on the creative aspect of this overlapping transitional playground as the root of our creativity, but it is difficult to describe this amorphous area of human experience in terms of affect, what being in it and sharing with other feels like. When you are trying to evoke elusive experience you need to avoid foundering on the twin rocks of sentimentality and nebulous subjectivity. Just because we are giving our minds free rein does not mean we cannot observe what is happening. We may have suspended our boundaries but we are not drifting helplessly.

What does the experience of sharing a creative playground actually feel like? The more we try to pin it down in words, the more it has a tendency to slither away. It is resistant to crystallisation. So I am going to approach it obliquely by borrowing from a different discipline, from the description of an exhibition of abstract paintings of luminous beauty by an artist called Hugonin. The art critic Lubbock writes (2002): '...though it asks nothing but looking...and is made with perfect ocular pitch and is so light sensitive...I'm not even sure that it is inherently a visual art. Its means are visual...[but] *what it offers is a structure of experience, a form of intense though calm attention, which involves change and continuousness, without repetition and without conclusion – and this is something the mind can find in looking, or equally in some kinds of reading or thinking. But however it happens, it takes as long as you've got*'.

The review continues by comparing the paintings with those in another exhibition: 'Both bodies of work have a penumbra of spirituality which may be another word for dedicated attention.'

In other words, through what I have referred to previously as 'intimate attention' (Caldwell 2000), it is possible to move beyond the particularities of an immediate shared sensory experience (in the example above, a visual experience shared with the painter) to a place where the mind wanders, reciprocally moved and moved on by what we discover in those we share with – and what they and we uncover in ourselves. What I experience in terms of feeling is awareness without interpretation, a deep stillness combined with wonder.

Referring back to Donna Williams in *Autism and Sensing* (1998), this is more than merging. The mind does not actually identify with 'other': on the borderlines of consciousness it is aware of self and what self is doing. One might call it a state of reciprocal induction, 'as it is' but also 'in the presence of', non-judgemental, active in the sense of awareness and response, passive in the sense of floating rather than swimming. As the reviewer says, it takes as long as you've got.

To return to earth, attention is on the particularities of what we are doing but is also on, or 'in,' the partner with whom we are sharing the sensory experience, whatever it is. What is evident when you enter this wandering state of mutual response is how much pleasure it gives both parties involved. While I do not wish to project my feeling onto the person with whom I am working, this sense of tranquillity and wonderment is characteristically present and can be observed and recorded (Caldwell, 2002).

What relevance does this rather philosophical approach have? Does it matter if we know what we are doing and who we are?

It is important not because we need to endlessly dwell on ourselves but so that we can be as present as possible to the people whose attention we are trying to engage, and also so that we avoid if possible projecting our own feelings on to them. If we know ourselves better, next time we are at the sharp end of a tantrum we will be more aware of all the issues involved. We will be able to distinguish between our feelings and those of the person who is upset, between our fear and their despair, pain, frustration or anger. We will understand a little more that the person's outburst is not personally directed but arises from her inability to handle the situation in which she finds herself. Under the circumstances she is in, she is overwhelmed by her defensive reactions to a situation she finds intolerable.

Even more important, it moves beyond disability and is something we both give and receive. It values the other person and the feeling that he or she is valued empowers them. They are able to give as well as receive. This is the equality that we talk about so much.

When they respond to our overtures we need to welcome them, drawing them into all the possibilities of creative relationship in a way that is safe for them. At the same time, we need to trust them and allow ourselves to be drawn into their creative sphere. If all this sounds complicated it is only because it is helpful to reflect sometimes on an ideal state. But we are none of us perfect. What we can do is to be aware of pitfalls. We can relax, lay aside our own preoccupations and suppositions, look and listen with intent and, to borrow a phrase from Winnicott, be 'good enough' (1971).

The next question I want to address is not so much a developmental one, how this consciousness of self arose, but what happens if this goes wrong: if I have failed to develop a sense of my singularity or if, having developed it, the sense of self is displaced. How can this happen?

I am informed by the feedback from my external and internal senses. If all is going well there is constant free trade between my brain, body and the world out there, telling me what I am doing and adjusting my responses. Problems arise if my sensory experience is so erratic that the boundary that helps me to define myself fails to develop, is amorphous, or if it has become a barrier. In one case I am not able to properly separate myself from the world out there so I do not recognise 'other'. Alternatively, the boundary is present but because of its solidity I am not able to reach out from 'my world' to 'the world'.

This may be the outcome of physical limitation. If one or more of my senses is deficient I shall have an additional struggle and must rely on extra sensitivity and training of the remaining senses to reach and be reached by the world outside. But it can also be that, having approached the world outside, my experience of it is just too scary to handle. I retreat back into my inner world where I feel less threatened. Then, since I am cut off from the world outside, my overwhelming sensory experience is derived from my internal feedback. I focus all my attention on a particular sensation, to the exclusion of everything else. I scrape the grain of the wood or scratch the fabric of my chair with my fingernail and listen to the sound it makes. I am completely absorbed and may even identify my sense of self with this activity.

Under these circumstances my retreat back into my inner world may be total. In the Channel 4 film Jam Jar: An Inside-Out Approach, Donna Williams describes how, when she found the demands of the world too frightening, she withdrew from relationships. She explains that all the relationships she should have had with the people out there she made with the shadowy world inside. She illustrates this by using glass beads as people. She sorts them into related pairs and groups according to their properties and says: 'Everybody knows who they are in relatedness to everybody else. But what if the knowing really scares you? What if the knowing doesn't give you a good knowing? What if the knowing doesn't tell you, you have a brother or cousin? What if the knowing tells you that you are not at all related to anybody and the best you can do is be an impostor in that other solar system?'

Gunnilla Gerland describes her isolated world: 'I spent a great deal of time inside myself, as if in my own world screened off from everything else. But there was no world there inside me, nothing more than a nothing layer, a neither-nor, a state of being hollow without being empty or filled without being full. It just was, in there, inside myself. I was inside the emptiness and the emptiness was inside me – no more than that. It was nothing but a kind of extension of time. I was in that state and it just went on' (Gerland, 1996).

Where can we meet someone who feels herself to be alone, 'living in an alien world', as an unidentified child with ASD put it in the Radio 4 broadcast A Bridge of Voices; someone who simply does not recognise the body language and interactive systems that bind us into friendships and relationships, with all their possibilities? If you want to meet me you are going to have to come to the front door of my sensory experiences. This is where I am.

Where shall we meet?

But before we try to meet we need to look at the psychological preconditions for such an encounter. One of the questions put to me at one of my workshops is: 'Do you empty yourself when you work?'

The answer to this question has to be 'yes and no': 'yes' in the sense that I try to lay aside my preoccupations, expectations, theories and projections, and 'no' in the sense that I have to be present to react and respond to the person with whom I am working. They will not be interested in empty air. I have to offer them myself, because this is the most valuable thing I have.

To say 'I am here for you' is to be completely open, to shed our defensive shells. To be 'I', present in the place of 'me' and simultaneously in the presence of other, is not only to be vulnerable, it is also opportunity. Here we can meet 'not-me' (other) in ways that are not possible while we are dug in behind our protective ramparts.

Another questioner says: 'Do you go in with a welcoming face and open body language?' Looking at video of myself, I wonder why I do not and realise that what is uppermost is intense concentration. Apart from the fact that to assume the person I am working with would perceive, for example, a smile as welcoming and not threatening, that their sensory perception occupies the same territory as mine, I need to put aside what I want to do with them and focus with all my attention on what they are doing so that I notice the tiniest movement and the smallest sound and, particularly, changes in these. What I am doing is looking for what has meaning to them, so I can respond to that rather than make assumptions about how we will relate. It is through sharing our selves and exploring each other in mutually creative ways that we are empowered.

When I am asked why we don't just leave people where they are, I have to reply it is not just that those accounts we have of living in the inner world paint it not only as a refuge but also as a prison. This can be lonely and scary. It also misses out on the positive enrichment offered by social interaction. Human beings are not programmed to be solitary animals. Even those who feel they wish to live on their own are totally dependent on the infrastructure of the society in which they exist. We cannot assume that the aloneness of those with disability is voluntary. 'People with ASD do have feelings. I do feel lonely' (Jolliffe *et al*, 1992).

We cannot, and would not wish to, force social contact on those who choose not to engage. What we can do is offer a means of enrichment in terms that are acceptable, and usually welcomed because they are non-threatening, to people whose world is scary and who do not have the intellectual resources of those who are high functioning. Those who are low functioning cannot find their way out of the maze on their own so they retreat into an interior life. They do not have the freedom to choose. When a high-functioning autistic person says 'I like myself as I am', this implies a considerable degree of self-knowledge and self-esteem.

Relationship is not a possibility for those whose disability is more severe. However the capacity for enjoying warm and loving interaction is not a function of intellectual ability; anyone can be enriched by it. What is very noticeable is that when a person starts to shift their attention from solitary self-stimulation to sharing their world, their whole demeanour and body language alters. They relax and begin to smile; they are able to give eye contact, interact by holding out their hands and may offer a hug – this even from people who normally find physical contact distressing and avoid touch. Stress is reduced to the extent that some will, of their own accord, start to use relevant words. It is clear that they want to communicate. The world is no longer seen as a hostile place but one that they so often choose to be in. This change can be dramatic.

Vera has no sight. She was 16 when staff were first shown how to use her sounds to talk to her. At the time she was banging her head so badly that she had to wear a helmet for self-protection and the home was also considering padding the walls with foam. Two years later her mother, who had described the increasing difficulties of containing Vera's wild behaviour both at school and at home and was present at the first session, says: 'You could see the change in her from the day people started using Intensive Interaction. After about five minutes she relaxed and became a different person and that is how she has stayed since then.' Vera no longer wears a helmet. Staff use her sounds as a way of talking to her and letting her know they are around all the time. She won best pupil award at school last year.

When I start to work with someone new, particularly if they have ASD, I may often wonder how on earth I am ever going to get close to them. It is not so much that I feel rejected; I feel simply ignored. I am not part of their world. But in order to learn to trust each other we have to meet in the sense that we need not only to observe their affective space – how they feel – but also to allow the other person to come into our space, where we are feeling and responsive. The prerequisite is proximity, getting it right in both the physical and psychological sense. We have to get close to each other in a way that feels right for both of us. We need to learn how to come and go in ways that are both respectful and fun.

Unfortunately there is no agreement that we should meet. When we start to try to engage the people with whom we are working they have not consented to the encounter. We have to go camouflaged, to slip in under cover of their language so they begin to enjoy the encounter before being alerted to possible danger. We need to get in under their defences without triggering alarm. We have to look for the feedback they are giving themselves because it is through this doorway of sensation that we shall be able to make contact. This is where they are. We will meet when their brain recognises something familiar. This will obtain low level attention from them. As explained in Chapter One, in order to move on to engagement we may have to add an element of surprise.

The ways in which we can do this are endless. It may simply be an infiltration of the way the person is talking to himself through feedback and sensations, but if the person is deeply withdrawn or afraid our overtures may also have to be sufficiently interesting to draw their attention away from their distress. We may need to climb over the fence while they are not looking.

A speech therapist is working with Richard, who is very afraid. If people come near him he makes noises of distress. As he becomes more threatened these rise almost to a bellow. She returns his sounds. This is not very effective until she starts ending them with a smacking sound made with taut lips. There is a look of amazement on his face as he turns to her with a radiant smile.

When we are working with people who have some speech we can be misled into thinking they are trying to communicate with us when sometimes they may be using words as a barrier behind which to hide. Very often it is not so much what they say as how it sounds. We need to listen to the tone of the voice. Is it free-running and flexible or tense with anxiety? Does it sound unattached? Characteristically, an individual who is using speech to protect himself will speak in the third person, often in a high-pitched, rather monotonous way. Their speech will sound flat, lacking in colour, modulation or change in tempo.

Sometimes the phrases people use reflect what has been said to them. You can almost hear the condemnatory tones of the original speaker in the words: 'Silly noises, stupid faces!'

The more able the person is, the more sophisticated the avoidance systems may be. In *Nobody Nowhere* (1992) Donna Williams describes how she adopted a variety of characters, each with their own voice, to survive particular situations that were otherwise intolerable. Recordings of her voice in each situation sound completely different; the change in quality of voice is very noticeable. Her most extraordinary achievement is that, even though she has severe ASD, she has also been able to learn to speak at least sometimes with her true voice, from her innermost self, without defence systems. This is something all of us need to learn.

The ability to relate to each other moves us from solitude to the possibilities of sharing, having friends and allies and being able to love.

Chapter Seven

MORE TO SEEING THAN MEETS THE EYE

- The quality of attention
- Tuning in
- The byways of capturing attention
- Pattern recognition
- Pointing the way – opening out

This section turns again to what we mean by the quality of 'attention', looking at a range of different ways of gathering it. This is not simply to create a longer list but to help explore some of the byways it leads us into. It is both about the focus of the person with whom I work on whatever it is that is the centre of their interest and what it means to them – and the essential focus that I must have on them.

Tuning in

If there is a tune on the radio we particularly want to listen to, we either turn up the volume or pay closer attention. We cut out extraneous noises and fine-tune our attention until we don't just hear, we listen with intent. If we really care about it we search and research the airwaves, moving closer to and becoming more and more involved in the source.

Attention is at the centre of our ability to engage: not just passing awareness but through sustained focus. We move from low-level attention to consciousness so that we begin not just to do something but to know what we are doing.

We are all capable of carrying on with behaviours of which we are not aware. A student swings his leg throughout a morning workshop. Near the end he says: 'I don't really know what you mean by repetitive behaviours.' He is quite unconscious of the low-level conversation going on between his brain telling the appropriate muscles in his leg to contract and relax and the feedback his brain is receiving in the form of what is presumably positive sensation, telling his brain that his leg has moved.

As our brains and bodies talk to each other we can listen either with low-level or focused attention. Moving into consciousness, we become the observers of ourselves – and also of our activities with objects (or people) that (or whom) we can modify, or be changed by. These objects with which we interact and the feelings that we draw from our interactions tell us both that we are and what we are doing. In Damasio's words: 'With consciousness there is the presence of "you" in a particular relationship to some object. The simplest form of such presence is the kind of image which constitutes a feeling – the feeling of what happens when your being is modified by the acts of apprehending something. The presence must be there or there is no you. Consciousness is the unified mental pattern that brings together the object and self' (Damasio, 1999).

So when I attend to continually using my forefinger to scrape the fabric of my chair, I engender a sense of self. Those of us who live in an ordered and reasonably predictable environment can only begin to guess how critical this is for a person whose world is constantly falling apart. Both the films A is for Autism and Jam Jar try to show us what are the actual physical effects experienced by people with ASD. In the first, a small boy shows us squiggly lines, constantly on the move, retreating particularly when he tries to focus on them. He tells us that the more he tries to concentrate on them the more they run away. Under these circumstances we cannot overestimate the importance of recognisable pattern, some theme, anything familiar to grab hold of in a chaotic world, anything to which the brain can relate.

Andy touches the skirting with his foot as he walks. This is seen as kicking. Another interpretation is that, in a world where he cannot rely on the visual sensory information regarding dimension and direction, he needs to reassure himself with the sense he does have, that of touch, as to the constancy of the line between the wall and the floor. Because it wriggles, he needs to know where it is and where he is in relation to it.

Thirty years ago when I was beginning to understand the need to find out what is important for a person in order to gain their attention, I was asked by a teacher if I could think of any way of helping a child with ASD and considerable behavioural problems that endangered other children.

Jennie is five. She attends school but cannot be engaged at all, except that she appears to be interested in reflected light flashing across the walls or ceiling: for example, the reflection from a piece of shiny metal. She becomes alert and follows it with interest. Otherwise she is cut off and occasionally hits other children. After some experimentation I make her a box with flanges that can be rotated horizontally on a frame. The surfaces are covered with styrene mirror in the hope that, as she turns the box to obtain the visual stimulus she enjoys, she may also start to look at herself. Her teacher works with Jennie every day. At first she just turns the box in order to see the light that bounces off it flit round the room. Gradually she spots and becomes more interested in her own image. In parallel, her aggression towards others decreases. Her attention has been drawn and engaged through the very specific stimulus that she recognises and enjoys.

However we need to be incredibly careful over presentation, since the stimulus that attracts one child may be dangerous for another. (In the case of the mirror box this is particularly important since it became a popular piece of equipment in special schools, where it is still sometimes used just as a general way of persuading a child to engage in anything and without thought for particular intention.) An occupational therapist reports the history of a child with epilepsy who puzzled care staff because every time they gave her a bath she had a seizure. They could not understand why until the therapist suggested that the origin of the problem might be reflected white light coming off the surface of the water.

Sandra refuses to have a bath because there is a snake in it. It is suspected that she is hallucinating until her carer bends down and looks at the water from the level at which Sandra sees it. The reflection of an overhead strip-light wriggles like a serpent on the surface of the water. The same stimulus of reflected light that was a doorway for one child proves to be a quite different type of trigger for others.

It is not always essential to present the particular stimulus that catches a person's attention in the same way as they are giving it to themselves. Very often they will recognise a familiar rhythm or pattern that underlies their self-stimulus.

Such pattern recognition can be visual or auditory or tactile, and can be represented in a different mode to that in which the themes were originally expressed.

Micky sits in a chair turning the dial on a toy telephone. He is unresponsive to approaches until I move my finger in a circle on the back of his hand, following the movements of his dial back and forwards as he does it. He smiles and pays attention.

Sue demonstrates a similar recognition of related pattern. She is in a class of more able children with ASD and disrupts their work with noises and generally chaotic behaviour, which it is difficult to get past. Among a number of repetitive behaviours it emerges that she likes to spend time twirling a windmill. She is immediately interested and focuses on my forefinger when I rotate it in the air in a similar fashion.

Rod is very difficult to make contact with and has very disturbed behaviour. He has no sight but he licks his lips in a circular manner. When I move my thumb round on the top of his foot in time to echo the movements of his tongue he becomes very attentive and laughs so loudly that it can be heard all over the house. Staff come running in. They have not heard him laugh before.

On the other hand Betty recognises the rhythm of her action when the wall is banged in time to her head banging.

Each time it was the pattern that was recognisable: an underlying pattern or theme that related to the sensory feedback the person was giving herself. I was confirming for the individual what she was doing and at the same time affirming her to herself. But I had also broken into the stereotypic sensory loop and was opening out what had been a closed situation. From now on there were other possibilities because her attention was able to move through territory that was familiar (and therefore safe) but also held the potential for new exploration. A behaviour that had been unconscious or semi-conscious was now fully conscious and, because we trusted each other, we could do things together without the risk that had kept the stereotypic behaviour going up until then. She could safely look out of the door; our attention now overlapped in the transitional playground. Our activity was joint-funded; we could explore together, sharing our delight and pleasure at each new innovation.

Through attention we move from seeing to looking, from looking to careful watching and from touching to feeling and conscious exploration. From passive participation we move into trust and from here into the endless creative possibilities of 'What if ?' .

Pointing the way

There are times when the people with whom we are working take very specific steps to point us towards ways of helping them to escape their repetitive loop. This is particularly true of people who are verbal, and it is absolutely critical that we listen very carefully to what they have to say.

Cassie, who has ASD, has occasional violent outbursts that start with her asking if you know about the number seven. This is a warning shot across the bows. From there on she builds into a tantrum over which she has no control and which presents dangers to those around her. During the build-up she actually says: 'The number seven is important!,' drawing our attention to the centre of her storm. When I use this to refocus her attention back into our world by asking if she is going to make seven sandwiches for her supper (an activity at which she was engaged at the time), she turns away laughing: 'No, I'm going to have three,' and goes back to getting her supper ready.

Even at the height of her storm, when the adrenalin was flowing freely, Cassie's brain took the lure. She was able to switch off and return to this world – but it was she who had already told me where she was in terms of where the 'core' was that was fuelling her frightening outburst.

There is a difference between this scenario and that of diverting attention. In diversion the person's attention is directed away from the subject to another, whereas in refocusing it is the subject itself that is removed from the inner to the outer world by changing its context.

In terms of letting us know how to help him, Jeff is even more explicit.

Jeff does not like to have a bath. He can be difficult when asked to do so for reasons of hygiene. However in his mind he has a girlfriend, a different one each week, and it is important that we know her name and keep up with his current favourite. One day his care worker was trying very hard to get him into the bathroom and eventually said, out of pure desperation: 'Maybe your girl friend would like you to have a bath so that you are nice and clean.' Jeff repeated it back to him: 'Yes, maybe my girl friend Mary would like me to have a bath so that I am nice and clean.' Thereafter whenever his care worker wanted him to have a bath they would go through this routine dialogue, but it only worked if the care worker inserted the name of the particular girlfriend of the week. If he got it wrong or failed to say a name, Jeff would correct him and say: 'Yes maybe my girlfriend Janice (or whoever it was that day) ... ' He would then wait for his key-worker to accept the prompt and repeat the sentence with the right name included. Then he would go off and have a bath. From being totally hostile to the idea of a bath he had become ambivalent: the idea of being clean for his girlfriend outweighed his distaste for washing. But he would make absolutely sure he obtained the release to let him out of his quandary by directing his care worker to use the proper word.

In this case it was if Jeff selected the right key from a bunch and thrust it under his care worker's nose, saying: 'Here's the right one. Use this to let me out.'

Tom, who has ASD, asks his mother when it is suppertime and she replies, 'Soon'. He bursts out: 'You know I can't manage soon!' but calms down at once when she says 'Six minutes'. In this case the distress is not about the repetitive loop. Tom is telling his mother that he cannot understand an abstract concept such as 'soon'. Although he can say it the word has no meaning attached to it and throws his brain into confusion.

All the above situations underline the importance of really taking on board the reality experienced by the person with whom we work.

Chapter Eight

WHO'S AFRAID OF WHOM?

- Fear as an ingredient of relationship
- Fear as part of a defence mechanism
- Fear of inadequacy
- Fear of not knowing what will happen

Working with people with severe learning disabilities – and particularly those with ASD – we sometimes come across people whose behaviour is such that we are at a loss how to relate to them. They may have outbursts, during which they may harm themselves and those who live with them and threaten us, sometimes to the point of injury. We are afraid. We feel we cannot cope. We do not like to talk about it in case others think we are inadequate. We feel they may laugh at us and we may be excluded from a team who appear to be managing. We exclude ourselves in order not to have to face the possibility of rejection by others.

What about the people we work with? The probability is that behaviours we see as challenging are the outcome of their also feeling afraid – part of their defence system against circumstances with which they cannot cope.

When this happens, fear becomes an ingredient of the relationship and this is a bad basis for interaction. We have to try to tease out what is really happening, who is afraid of whom and what are the roots.

'I spend my whole life being afraid, not just of what is happening now but also that something terrible may happen in the future' (Jolliffe, 1992).

'It got to the point where I was afraid of coming into work, not just because I might get hurt but also because I was afraid of being put in situations that I couldn't cope with.'

The first quotation is from a woman with ASD, describing the sensory distortions she experiences and what it feels like to exist in a reality where you are constantly afraid of the chaos and pain caused by various hypersensitivities. The second was said by a key worker, a young man, reflecting on a situation two years previously when the behaviour of the man he was looking after was extremely threatening, endangering both himself and those who cared for him. These quotations highlight the complex and diverse nature of fear, and in particular the part played by anticipation and the stress that this can cause. Fear is not just about what is happening now but what may happen in the future.

Roots run deep

'Irrespective of the fact that our ability to feel scared probably developed independently from our capacity to deal with danger, being afraid is the emotionally visible part of a defence mechanism which ensures our survival. Interactions between the defence system and consciousness underlie feelings of fear – but the defence system's function in life is survival in the face of danger' (Le Doux, 1998).

We are dealing with primal stuff. It is normal to feel afraid when we feel we are entering a dangerous situation – and the people we work with sometimes come with the label 'DANGER' clearly tied to them. Quite often this refers to the outcome of inappropriate treatment they have received. As soon as you start to use the language that their brain recognises as non-threatening and therefore respectful, this distressed behaviour usually melts away. We have caused so much of what we perceive as challenging.

The difficulty is that we are not always very good at assessing the degree of danger. We may exaggerate it, particularly if we are in situations we find difficult to read or when we misread the extent of the threat because of blueprints we are carrying round that derive from previous experiences and are only superficially related to the current circumstances. Sometimes the danger is in our minds.

Drawing on my own experience to illustrate how easy it is to misread a situation, the first time I visited a hospital for people with severe learning disability I was scared, almost entirely because I had never met people with disability before and was unable to read the facial and bodily language of a man because of his particular disability. He turned out to be the most gentle person.

(For me, one childhood blueprint still evokes an irrational but recognisable fear of walking through woods, which relates to the terrible fate of Red Riding Hood, Babes in the Wood etc. It always seemed to happen in the forest. Despite the fact that my rational brain is not deceived, wolves and ogres live on. They colour my current emotional responses.)

Our instinctive reactions to danger are those of avoidance, immobility, aggression or submission, responses with which we are all probably familiar in our daily lives. We need to be aware of what our own feelings are, because an aggressive response to a threatening situation will almost certainly make it worse.

People sometimes come with labels tied to them spelling 'DANGER' and reputations that frequently stem from previous inappropriate care. It is easy to allow this to dominate our feelings about them. But the astonishing thing is that as soon as you start to engage with them respectfully and use the language their brain recognises, their aggression begins to melt away.

Damasio (1994) points out that *if we are conscious of our emotional responses, feeling our affective states offers flexibility*. We can make choices about how we respond to a given situation. We do not have to respond instinctively. Instead we can look at ourselves, how we dealt with the fear that was triggered as part of our defence mechanism. As well as asking how we deal with the circumstances when we are attacked, we need to enquire what triggered the outburst. For example, it is very tempting to try to adopt the position of total control, putting the lid on and sitting on it. When I was trying to work with someone who had what was called 'difficult behaviour', a young man said to me: 'I don't know why you bother. He sits down if I shout at him.'

What he did not understand was that it was precisely his extreme attitude that was causing the stress that triggered the outburst in the first place. The same danger lurks in some behavioural practices if they are applied in ways that increase stress rather than promote tranquillity. We need to look not just at immediate containment but at why people are distressed.

Turning to our own fear, the key worker whom I quoted at the beginning of this section was quite rightly afraid of being hurt but he also said that he was afraid of not being able to cope. This is quite a common sensation if we are working with someone who is very difficult. (In this case the man he was working with had a tendency to strip off in public places, a situation that is very difficult to handle. What do you do about it? Sitting down in the middle of the road to persuade them may not be an option on a busy highway and a stand-up struggle is an equally unsuitable strategy.) The feeling of being inadequate to the situation is accompanied by the suspicion that others could have managed better and that you will be laughed at by colleagues. This leads directly into the life-threatening situation of feeling 'excluded'. We feed off primitive feelings. For our ancestors rejection from the pack could be a life sentence; no wonder we are afraid. But it is taboo to admit that you are afraid. Which is why leadership and team working are so vitally important. We must always be positive in our support of each other, for the most basic reason that we can help each other from sliding down the emotional slippery slope occasioned by fear.

At the same time we have to address the reasons why the person we are working with feels the need to attack us or to behave in an anti-social manner. What are they trying to tell us?

To illustrate this I am going to tell at length Jessie's story.

Jessie is 29. While there are many positive sides to her character she also used to have frequent and severe behavioural outbursts, causing injury to staff. It got to the point where people were extremely reluctant to work with her. Jessie lives in her own flat supported by a one-to-one service. I visit her both at her flat and at the resource centre and afterwards have a discussion with her support team, during which the following points arise. In spite of her behaviour, which is sometimes extremely difficult to manage, Jessie is an affectionate lady who loves to be told she looks good. She really thrives on positive personal input. She has a terrific sense of humour and likes people to be polite to her and say 'Please' and 'Thank you'. Although there are some features of her behaviour that could be seen as autistic, such as her desperate need for control and when she gets stuck in the middle of tasks, her sense of fun and ability to size people up suggest that her autism, if it is such, is not entirely typical.

When I first saw her, it was clear that Jessie had very poor self-esteem. In common with people who have this problem, her threshold for feeling threatened was extremely low and she reacted accordingly. The way staff had worked with her, giving her very close attention, had resulted in a marked improvement in her difficult behaviour during the last four years. There were fewer outbursts, although when these occurred they were serious. Outbursts were more likely to occur at the centre than at home. Staff could not tell what was going to trigger her off. They felt it was usually unpredictable. During her outbursts she was liable to kick, thump, rip and also hit walls. (When we label an outburst unpredictable it means that we have not been able to link it to a cause yet. We need to go on looking: outcome may be separated from cause, as in emotional overload. When this happens the response is delayed and separated by time from the cause (Williams, 1996).)

We held a large group meeting with all the people involved in Jessie's care to try to tease out what was really going on. It emerged through discussion that most of her distressed behaviour occurred if she felt she was losing control, particularly when she was working on a one-to-one basis and a third person came and interrupted. The actual point at which she became distressed was when her one-to-one worker turned away to address the needs of the incomer. It seemed to me that up until that time she knew what she was doing but as soon as she lost contact with what was going on she was projected into what was, for her, chaos. Considering this, we came up with the following guidelines.

- Jessie needs to feel herself to be in control.
- Jessie needs to know what is going to happen before it happens so she has time to think about it. (When we discussed this, staff said that they thought they had been

doing this by giving her choices. What they had not realised was the need to break down everything they did with Jessie into small stages that she could grasp and get her assent to each stage.) If she says 'No' we need to accept it, so that she can run her own life in a way that she understands.

- She does not like it if other people come between her and the person with whom she is engaged. She finds it very difficult to wait.
- She cannot cope with change.

With people like Jessie you cannot over-emphasise the need for a negotiating attitude, as opposed to a control attitude. It has been pointed out to me by clinical psychologist Pete Coia that negotiation is successful when both parties are happy with the conclusion. In Jessie's situation the agreement must be heavily weighted towards her being in charge of what happens. Above all, Jessie needs to know what is going to happen before it happens, so she has time to take it on board. You can see her thinking about it when you tell her something. Explain and wait until she indicates by a nod that she has understood. You may have to tell her more than once. She responds well to negotiation, which gives her control. At the centre, if people come up and talk to the person with whom she is working, it is suggested that they turn to her before engaging the other person and say, 'Jessie, I need to sort this out. I'll be back with you in a minute. All right?' If they can get her permission before turning away, giving her time to agree, this gives her the control she so badly needs. She knows they will come back. As a result of using this technique, her outbursts have declined dramatically.

Another strategy staff have adopted is to telephone Jessie before she leaves her flat to let her know what she is going to do when she arrives at the centre. This works very well. She will now pick up the phone and answer it herself.

If it turns out that staff cannot comply with Jessie's wishes for reasons beyond their control, the way they lay down the boundary is critical; she must have time to process the change so that she is not faced with a sudden event which will activate her life-threatened response. To avoid this situation, if there is a change in plan while she is on her way to the centre, they use her escort's mobile to warn her. She never arrives at the centre without knowing what is going to happen.

To keep a person's attention they need to be highly motivated. For this reason it was suggested that on-site activities with Jessie in the centre should be based on things she most enjoyed doing, which would win reinforcing praise from others and make it easier to engage her. This would particularly include make-up sessions and attention to her hair, using a mirror to get her to look at herself. While Jessie finds a large mirror difficult, she will look at herself in a hand mirror.

Jessie's sense of humour, coupled with her love of being addressed politely, can be used to help her when she gets stuck. We cannot assume this is voluntary; sometimes the brain just will not issue the necessary instructions. In order to start her off again we may need to give clues in another mode. Elaborate over-politeness makes her laugh and she can then resume whatever she was doing.

Jessie would sometimes become distressed and have to be taken home from the centre. I suggested saying to her in the car, before she got home: 'I'm going to leave you in the flat so you can cool off. When you feel better, come and give me a knock in the office. OK?' This strategy gives her time to think about it before she gets home and also gives back to her some control by letting her decide how long the break should be.

Jessie is apt to tap people and they can find this irritating. In the past, no distinction had been made between this sometimes slightly inappropriate way of getting attention or exercising her sense of humour and when she hit someone. The staff needed to make sure they all reacted in the same way as some staff were still telling her it was bad to hit. Observation suggested that Jessie got quite a kick out of being told it was bad to hit; her tapping was having the effect she wanted and so she usually persisted. A better strategy seemed to be to make it into fun, to tap her very gently on the arm. This made her laugh and she might do it once more but quickly stopped. The same strategy proved helpful when she banged things.

Jessie has certain distinctive body movements, such as an upward and outward movement of her hands. While I did not feel specifically that Intensive Interaction would improve her ability to communicate, which was already extremely good, I found it helpful to incorporate her gestures into my own speech as a way of expressing solidarity with her and possibly increasing her attention.

While Blackburn, quoted in the Introduction, describes how her anxiety stems from the unpredictability of behaviour, some people may feel that we have gone over the top by letting Jessie know exactly what is happening all the time. However, giving her control, accepting it if she says 'No', works. Her agenda is more important than ours. Her outbursts have more or less ceased. From staff feeling unable to work with her, they now feel confident and clearly enjoy working with her.

Jessie was afraid and because they were getting hurt and unable to figure out what was wrong, so were the people who worked with her. We were able to help her and move her on by isolating the root causes of her distress. She is no longer afraid and nor are the people who work with her.

One of the main problems is that, when we are afraid, techniques to control behaviour are liable to add to the stress which a person is experiencing and increase rather than decrease the 'challenges' the person presents, even if they are channelled into another route. Control is not enough. We must address the fears and needs that underlie the person's outbursts.

When we are afraid we need to look at whether our fears are real and relate to actual situations or if they are the trailers of trauma in our earlier life. If they are real we need to search and research the possible causes of a person's distressed behaviour because the most probable one is that they are afraid. We always need to support each other.

CONCLUSION

- Building a relationship through shared exploration
- Learning to listen
- The relationship – what does it mean for both of us?

It is very easy to fall into the trap of thinking when we work with people with learning disabilities that we are the teachers. Although we talk about 'valuing people' we tend to assume that we are the ones who give, they receive. We talk about equality but do not behave as if we have anything to learn from them. We do not 'listen', in the sense of paying attention to what they are saying to us.

The successful infant needs to learn the skill of making friends. This is a biological imperative that helped us to survive when we lived in groups in what was basically a hostile environment. We still use it to improve the quality of our lives. Friendless, we are vulnerable and lonely. We need allies to support us and we make these by sharing the things we enjoy, in the hope that our prospective friend will also enjoy them. We are trying to engage their attention with the things we value. The process by which we make friends is by offering and accepting shared interests. To do this involves making ourselves vulnerable to the savage pain of rejection (which may have life threatening implications in the biological sense).

But there is a difficulty when trying to get in touch with people with ASD. We very often make the mistake of thinking that, because they do not show emotion, they do not feel it. Jolliffe (1992) tells us this is not so, that she is able to love and feel lonely. The problem for the person with ASD is that they cannot always handle the emotional feedback they get from their own nervous system, which may be painful for them. So they learn to avoid emotional contact. However, my experience is that if you use 'their language' and present it in a way that respects their hypersensitivities so that they do not find it painful, they frequently respond with warmth and a desire for contact. They will hug you, look you in the face, smile and show all the warmth one does for a friend.

We need to look at how it is they read the world – what is it that has meaning for them.

Gabriel has very severe autistic spectrum disorder and learning disabilities, with the additional complication of epilepsy. He is non-verbal and is locked into a world of repetitive self-stimulation such as flicking bundles of string or leaves or the close scrutiny of beads and gloves, especially rubber gloves. Staff say they feel cut off from him, cannot reach him, do not know what they should be trying to do since he responds to very little outside his own intimate world and pays little or no attention to activities he is offered. Sometimes he is extremely disturbed, crashing round the room and banging himself, particularly if he wants something he cannot have, although what this is may not be evident. Eventually he will calm down. At other times he is very sleepy – which may be partly caused by his anti-convulsants or, possibly, a disturbed sleep rhythm, which is not uncommon in people with ASD.

When Gabriel flicks a bead on a string (or pursues any of his repetitive behaviours) 'he knows what he is doing.' Here is a sensation with which his brain is familiar, that is recognisable and non-threatening. It is, so to speak, 'hard-wired' in. By focusing on this specific activity he can lock out chaos. Repetition produces calming endorphins, the 'feel-good' factors of the brain. But the intensity of his inward concentration cuts out his capacity to exchange with the world outside. It excludes interaction. He holds us at bay by pursuing activities that feed his inner world and protect him from what he perceives as harmful.

For us, a bead is just a bead – but if we look at it through the eyes of someone with ASD, we learn to explore a world of enhanced sensory perception. The bead has colour that changes in the light. It also has shape, weight density, texture and movement as it flicks, and sound on impact. We begin to explore another way of understanding the world through what Donna Williams in Jam Jar calls 'the world of sensing uncomplicated by the need for interpretation'. Through attention and joint exploration we start to learn to explore our sensory world in a way we may never have been able to before: a world of touch and feel, the world of here and now unclouded by recollection of the past or anticipation of the future. If we will let them, the person with ASD will lead us further through the mysterious world of 'qualia', exploring the greenness of green, the tone of a sound and the muskiness of a rose, a sensory exploration in the transitional playground as yet unexplained in neurobiological terms.

For us, this adds an important dimension because we live in closed worlds. As infants we learned to cut out so much of our sensory world. We learned to choose what was good for us and exclude that which our brains decided was irrelevant. For example, if we stop what we are doing and listen we begin to hear what the world around us is doing: the business of traffic, clocks, bird song, electronic hums, the creaks of our house and the whispers of wind and rain; we hear sounds that may have no immediate relevance for us but which nevertheless exist in their own right.

Much of this sensory selectivity is necessary so that, in our complex world, we can concentrate on processing those events that do have meaning for us. The downside is that we learn to focus on ourselves; we live from our own needs, cutting our worlds down to the size of our own sensory reality. We call this 'our point of view' and base our judgements on our own realities, the scenarios that have worked for us. For example, when I walk into a room I may unconsciously make assessments based on that elusive quality known as 'taste', which comes down to whether or not I could share interests with the house's owner and therefore enjoy being friends with them. Would they make good allies? Whether I like it or not, I look at the world through the tinted lenses of my own perspective. How does this experience relate to me?

Through exploration of the enhanced sensory perception of the person with ASD we begin to move out of ourselves towards seeing the world as it is, uncluttered by our expectations. We begin to share in a world that is not based on our own needs. And, particularly, we start to be able to share fun, thereby completing the circle because it is through sharing fun that we most quickly make friends. By seeing the world through their eyes we are liberated, if only for a short time, from the burden of ourselves. We become for each other as we are.

What does our partner get out of it? In Jam Jar Donna Williams speaks of the war raging inside her that was set off by the difficulty of living in and conforming to a world that always insisted on her using a system based on attaching meaning and interpretation to sounds. Her brain worked directly from sensation. She describes a table as 'the flat brown lined thing' that 'impacted' with a certain thud when hit. She did not necessarily need to go on to call it 'table' or think, 'That's what you put the plates on'. While we may point out that it is difficult to generalise from this system, this was how she saw it and it worked for her. She was deeply stressed by people shouting at her that she was stupid and felt even more alienated from others.

In the same film, Williams speaks of the discovering the delight of discovering relationships, and illustrates it with video of herself and her friend Paul, who is also autistic. On the beach together they explore the sensation of the squelching sound their feet make in wet muddy sand. She comments: 'Now I can be, not just me in my world but me in my world and him in my world.'

The vast emptiness of a world lived in separateness is breached. She is no longer on her own; there is someone else with whom she can be a child and share fun.

When we work with someone with ASD they are allowing us to share something they value, and in the intensity of our mutual exploration there is nothing put on or phoney about the value we place on their gift and, by extension, on them. When we work with them in this way, both they and we cross the bridge out of ourselves and in our mutual absorption become 'WE'. This is what valuing a person really is: not some theoretical appreciation but being 'with' and 'in' and 'for' each other. Next time it will be easier. We will know that mutual attention to sensation can lead both of us to the art and joy of being together.

REFERENCES

Barron J., Barron S. (1992) *There's a Boy in Here*. New York: Simon and Schuster.

Blackburn R. (2002) Flint NAS seminar. 15 July.

Caldwell P. (1998) *Person to Person*. Brighton: Pavilion Publishing.

Caldwell P. (2000) *You Don't Know What It's Like*. Brighton: Pavilion Publishing.

Caldwell P. (2002) *Learning the Language*. Training video. Brighton: Pavilion Publishing.

Damasio A. R. (1994) *Descartes' Error: emotion, reason and the human brain*. New York: Grosset/Putnam.

Damasio A. R. (1999) *The Feeling of What Happens*. London: Heinemann.

Ephraim G. (1986) *A Brief Introduction to Augmented Mothering*. Radlett, Herts: Harperbury Hospital School.

Gerland G. (1996) *A Real Person*. London: Souvenir Press.

Greenfield S. A. (1997) *The Private Life of the Brain*. London: Allen Lane.

Hobson P. (2002) *The Cradle of Thought*. Basingstoke: Macmillan.

Jolliffe T., Lansdown R., Robinson C. (1992) Autism: a personal account. *Communication* **26** (3).

Le Doux J. (1998) *The Emotional Brain*. London: Weidenfield and Nicholson.

Lubbock T. (2002) Rich Creations of Patience. *The Independent* 2 July.

Moyles J. R. (1989) *Just Playing*. Buckingham: Open University Press.

Nadel J., Canioni L. (1993) *New Perspectives in Early Communicative Development*. London: Routledge.

Nafstad A., Rodbroe I. (1999) *Co-creating Communication with Persons with Congenital Deaf-Blindness*. Dronninglund, Denmark: Forlaget-Nord Press.

Nind M., Hewett D. (1994) *Access to Communication*. London: David Fulton Press.

Peeters T. (1997) *Autism: from theoretical understanding to educational intervention*. London: Whurr Publishers.

Rankin K. (2000) *Growing Up Severely Autistic: they call me Gabriel*. London: Jessica Kingsley Publishers.

Rodbroe I., Souriau J. (2000) Communication. In: McInnes J M (ed) *A Guide to Planning and Support for Individuals who are Deaf/Blind*. Toronto: University of Toronto Press.

Seybert J. (2002) Keynote speech. Maryland Coalition for Inclusive Education. 3 October. Maryland: Baltimore.

Williams D. (1992) *Nobody Nowhere*. London: Doubleday.

Williams D. (1994) *Somebody Somewhere*. London: Doubleday.

Williams D. (1996) *Autism: an inside-out approach*. London: Jessica Kingsley Publishers.

Williams D. (1998) *Autism and Sensing*. London: Jessica Kingsley Publishers.

Winnicott D. W. (1971) *Playing and Reality*. London: Tavistock Press.

Zeedyke S. (2002) Personal communication.